IT'S ALL ABOUT CANCER

A Personal Journey –

Help and Guidance for

Longevity and Prevention

Written by JULIE ROMANI

www.itsallaboutcancer.co.uk

Published by HERMIT MEDIA

England 2014

Published Jan 2014 by Hermit Media Ltd. PO Box 804,Haywards Heath, England, RH16 9LB

Printed by T J International Ltd. Trecerus Industrial Estate, Padstow, England, PL28 8RW

ISBN : 978-0-9927180-0-8

This book is dedicated to Joe Romani who was a loving husband to Julie and a devoted father to his children.

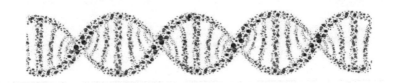

Contents Hermit

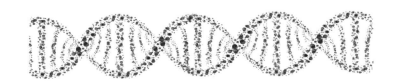

Foreword

This story would seem to be a story of 'failure', of a young man born in poverty who struggles to escape and, having succeeded, finds that he has developed a lethal cancer. He subsequently dies after spending as much of his wealth as he could trying unsuccessfully to outwit the cancer, using every conventional, and many unconventional, treatments which many people would never have the opportunity to afford.

As a person who had the privilege to be at the epicentre of this struggle and who sometimes disapproved of some of the treatments tried, I could only marvel at the indomitable spirit of the man. However, even more so, I came to respect the indomitable spirit of his wife, the author of this book who, with only a GCSE pass in biology, was able to analyse and debate with many experts whose work she researched and selected to try in her search for the cure.

This book focuses on the 'alternative' and research approaches which Julie adopted. Whilst none gave lasting results, which is understandable with such a late stage diagnosis, each had a degree of success and Joe survived nearly six years after failing surgery compared to the less than two predicted, until the final days experiencing life to the full.

Even now many of the newer drugs which Joe was prescribed, and particularly many of the 'alternative' therapies, have not been published in full and perhaps one lesson for the future is the need for more rapid methods to achieve earlier reporting of self–funded research. However, the real need is for greater attention to the positive messages about the role of regular exercise and sunshine in defending against cancer in anyone employed in a 'normal' full–time job in an urban environment (see *www.orchid-cancer.org.uk/738/Sport-&-Education*). This education process needs to begin in schools.

Equally important is for teachers to recognise pupils who aren't bookworms and channel their energies into activities that engage their latent practical skills and not just be obsessed by the three 'Rs' which should still be taught alongside these practical activities.

For patients, their partners and anyone interested in achieving a healthy lifestyle, this book will provide lasting inspiration and much practical advice on 'leaving no stone unturned' when researching health advice on the internet.

Kindly written by Professor Oliver

Most of my patients (about 70%) are oncological and come to me after being diagnosed, treated with chemo and radiotherapy and told that there is not much left to be done.

The outstanding situation with Joe Romani was the support which he had from his family, especially his wife Julie, who was lovingly reminding him (not pushing) regarding what treatments to do and what supplements to take — in fact she went so far down this path that she became an expert in nutrition and supplementation.

Joe did his best to fight against cancer, even purchasing some of the medical equipment which I use in my own clinic in order to receive home treatments. He knew how to enjoy life, be it sailing, eating, drinking or hanging out with friends. He even learned to enjoy his treatments, especially when he (along with his family) visited me in Spain.

It was very sad for me to lose Joe. Nevertheless his family and I are aware that we did all that was possible in order to help him to live well whilst he was with us. I wish that all of my patients were like Joe and all of the wives like Julie.

Kindly written by Dr Hilu

There is one thing that beats all medical treatments of cancer known to this day — the support of a loved one. Joe was lucky enough to have Julie, which in my opinion extended his life the biggest way.

Kindly written by Dr Seeger

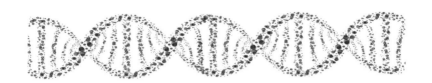

Acknowledgements

I would especially like to thank Professor Oliver for his unswerving help and support, together with Dr Seeger and Dr Hilu.

I would like to thank Emma Bonney for her editorial advice and my sister, Linda, for helping to make this book happen.

I would like to thank everyone who has kindly given permission for their inclusion in this book.

I would like to thank everyone who buys this book for their kind donation to Orchid Cancer Research.

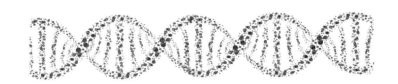

1 —About the Book

Three Little Words

'You have cancer'. There can be few sentences which have the power to halt with a thud every thought in your head, every breath in your lungs. Time stands still as the silent bubble enfolds you. Once the shock wears off and your brain makes sense of the words which have been spoken, the assault on your senses begins. You feel simultaneously angry, scared, cold, shaky, hot, tired, despondent, sad, defiant — and most of all alone, because this terrible, silent, unseen monster has chosen you to sneak up on, to take as its prey. Surely they have got it wrong, they have the wrong person; it can't be you.

So what is this 'c' word anyway? It is a disease of the genes, which are part of a human **DNA**. Many changes in the DNA are accidental. Cells constantly divide and each time that they do, they have to copy their genetic code completely. When this process takes place, which happens all day every day, sometimes mistakes happen and the replication isn't exact which results in altered cells. The immune system will destroy the majority of these altered cells, but sometimes some of these cells invariably escape, especially when the immune system is already impaired or weakened by some other underlying or undiagnosed imbalance or illness. Some changes wouldn't make very much difference to how the cell works, but this one change may take that cell one step further towards producing cancerous cells.

The most common cancers are cancers of the skin, lung, colon, breast (in women) and **prostate** (in men). Also prevalent are cancers of the kidneys, ovaries, uterus, pancreas, bladder and rectum. Blood and lymph node cancers, such as leukaemia, are also common. Cancer can be either primary or secondary. For example, a person can be diagnosed with breast cancer only to find that, when investigations take place, this is the secondary cancer, and the primary cancer was somewhere else in the body first and then spread to the breast.

Cancer would seem to be non–discriminatory, the luck of the draw. However, the risk of developing cancer increases as individuals age with sixty percent of all cancers being diagnosed in people who are over sixty five years of age. Lifestyle choices can also affect the risk factor. It can seem unjust that some people live totally unhealthy lifestyles and never get cancer whereas some people who have lived clean, healthy lifestyles fall victim. I wish that I could say that Joe, my husband, fell into the latter camp, but our lifestyle only became healthy in later life, even more so after the diagnosis.

No two cancers are exactly the same. Because of this it is difficult to treat one cancer in exactly the same way as another. Currently much effort is being invested in research to test individual drug sensitivities of patient's tumour cells, either those taken at the time of surgery or more commonly using new cell sorting techniques to sort cells circulating in the patient's blood. Though not standard of care in most cancers, it has enabled doctors to focus on a smaller list of potentially effective treatments. So far there is no evidence of long–term cure in most cancers using these techniques and more significantly there are difficulties in modelling drugs in combination. It is recognised as the way to go forward as the actual cost of testing each individual's sensitivity to the various chemotherapies and drugs is far cheaper than testing each drug in the patient. Already, in breast cancer, routine testing of diagnostic tissue for hormone sensitivity is undertaken and there are encouraging results from testing for genetic damage which indicate sensitivity to the drug Herceptin. In other cancers such as lung, prostate and colon, early results are promising for selecting which drugs not to use, although they are less successful with prospective selection because of the inability to predict toxicity.

Two underlying processes are responsible for causing most cancers. The first is failure to repair specific genetic damage to DNA caused by external (mostly environmental) factors and the second is a weak or inefficient immune system. When the immune system is weak it fails to recognise the wrongly formed cells and destroy them. It could already be busy and weakened due to other problems in the body, perhaps an ongoing viral infection, a bad tooth, too many toxins in the body, too much bad bacteria, so that attention is not given where it is needed to destroy the bad cells.

Some cancers are like forest fires when genetic damage is very advanced whilst other early cancers are like slow burning log fires. Every cancer is different, just as every patient is different.

Which brings me to the question — why am I writing this book?

Live or Let Die

My husband, Joe, was told those very words — 'you have cancer'. As his wife I was told those words too, for he was my life. One in three — they had never seemed bad odds until then.

After the initial shock, people react in various ways — the defeatist who is ready to give up there and then because it's just too much like hard work; the optimist who is certain that they beat cancer every day so they will also be fine; the God–fearing person who faithfully trusts God to do what is best for them; the angry person who blames the world for their bad luck. And the fighter.

Joe and I belonged to the latter camp — the fighters. Joe's diagnosis was about as bad as it could be — the cancer had already **metastasised** i.e. spread to other parts of the body, in this case the bones — and it was not a question of 'if' he would die but 'when'. Joe loved life and lived it to the full, and we were not about to let him just slip quietly away without putting up the best fight that we could. The battle was helped by the fact that, from the very beginning until quite near the end, Joe lived in denial. He refused to accept that he was truly ill because he had too much life left to live.

I never really thought about why people got cancer or what caused it until Joe was diagnosed. Then, as if dredged from some depths where the information had slept silently until the right time, I began to recollect articles and stories that I had read about how people had beaten cancer, or at least made the quality of life good for longer, with alternative therapies not available on the NHS or even readily available in the private sector in the UK. I knew that I couldn't save Joe as the diagnosis was terminal, but my head exploded with questions about how I might be able to keep him alive for longer, keep him with me. We were extremely fortunate in that money was no object, but all that our money could do was buy time for Joe, buy the knowledge to help him. So I would spend as much of it as was necessary to give my husband a year, two, three, who knew?

With a team effort which combined my continuous research and Joe's commitment to the cause we kept Joe alive for seven years after the diagnosis, with a good quality of life until a month before the end. This was five years longer than the prognosis.

The reason for writing this book is to share our journey with you in the hope that something, anything, which we learnt may help someone else to fight or prevent cancer. I know that Joe would feel that his death was not in vain if one person was helped by the information which I share here. At the very least, by reading this book you will know that someone has survived this terrible disease far longer than it wanted him to, and that you will have hope and comfort from a shared experience. When you lose your reason for living you must find another — my reason is not to let Joe's life be forgotten or the things that we learnt go to waste.

It is all too often the case that, following the death of a person, those closest often regret that they did not try other treatments and the key is to 'leave no stone unturned'. I can honestly say that I could not have tried anything more and I would not have taken a different path. I may have changed the timings of certain things, for example, I would have visited the Cancer Clinic for a second opinion before deciding on any chemotherapy, had I known about it sooner, because of their earlier adoption of laboratory testing of the tumour. I may also have been stricter with Joe if I could have ever believed that we would eventually lose our fight. But I never accepted the prospect of Joe dying.

I believe that we must try everything, fight it with every ounce of strength and determination, and then it can be beaten, or at least put to sleep for a while longer. Belief is the strongest weapon in the arsenal.

Simply changing one small thing a week could change your future health and longevity. This is my hope for you, just as it was a lesson for me. When I was younger I had a problem with my lungs. I was a smoker and my doctor told me that if I didn't stop smoking I would lose my beauty at an earlier age than I might otherwise. Being a vain individual who values her looks I immediately stopped smoking. I wanted something very badly so I did something about it. My aim is to pass on my findings in the hope that you might read something which will change how you live as a healthy person, or that it might provide renewed vigour if you are battling with cancer. Prevention is much better than cure so perhaps after reading this book you may contemplate accepting that you own your body and your health and you may make some valuable changes.

I am not a medical person, but I was able to make informed choices using my common sense based on facts, and by asking the right questions of the right people. The choices were not always the right choices — hopefully some small detail in this book might save someone from making the same mistakes that we made. Hopefully you will gain the confidence to ask the awkward questions which make you feel unsure, and not be forced to hand your life-choices to someone else.

At the end of the book is a glossary. Wherever I have used the name of a drug or a condition which is not explained in the body of the text (the name or word being in bold and underlined when first used), I have explained this in the glossary. (I have also added in brackets the most recognised brand name of the drug, but this does not signify that this is the only brand name). This ensures that each person has their own choice of how they choose to use this book, depending on what they wish to gain from reading it. Some people will want to skim over the detailed names and just read about the journey and the pitfalls, others will want to know the details of particular issues and not others, whilst some people will want to know everything. Hopefully, this format facilitates a personal experience. There is also an index listing the various treatments, supplements, diets and details which can be found in the book, ensuring that the information can be quickly located.

There are many drugs, treatments, supplements and cleanses described which we used in our fight. Some of these have been shown to be effective on animals and not humans (I make no ethical comment or distinction about testing on animals; that is not the purpose of this book). Some have been shown to be effective on humans but only in certain kinds of cancer and not others. I make no distinction in my analysis of how tried or tested any of these might or might not be. To do so would mean that constant updating would be needed as new drugs or treatments which are effective against the spread of cancer are being approved or discovered every day. As an example, I recently took a flight and had the privilege of sitting with an elderly lady who was being kept alive by a new drug which had only recently been discovered. Had this drug been approved six months from now she may have already been dead. As I sit writing this book a new drug is being offered to women at high risk of being diagnosed with breast cancer, a major breakthrough. So please bear this in mind when considering treatments.

Although I have carried out much research in many forms, in most cases I have not included web links and bibliography. Again, to so would require constant updating. However if, having read the book, you would like more information or details of research paths, then please contact me through the web site and I will be happy to help in any way that I am able.

Please also bear in mind that I am not a doctor of any description. My writings are based purely on the experiences which Joe and I shared and the decisions which we took based on my research. I do not offer advice, only information and personal opinion. Nothing contained in this book is intended to replace the advice given to you by your medical practitioner because one ultimately needs to have a team on hand to keep an overall eye on long–term care. Should you decide to try alternative treatments, I would strongly advise that this is only after consultation with them.

The purpose of this book is to provide information which will help you to discuss your body without feeling unable to question the advice being given, but **nothing** in this book is claiming to diagnose, cure, treat or prevent any disease, including cancer.

I hope that you enjoy the book and reading about our journey and our battle in the shadows of cancer. Most of all, I hope to pass on Joe's legacy; the will to live as long and fruitful a life as possible in a healthy, happy and informed way.

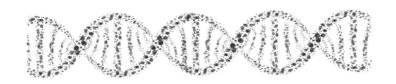

2 — Just a Man

For as long as he could remember Joe had dreamt about being a millionaire, whatever it took. At the age of twelve he put together his plan whilst sitting on the playing fields, watching a cricket match. He knew that he would be rich whichever way, by good means or bad. That became his only focus, with no concern as to where he might sleep, eat or live.

He hated his family home; it was filthy. Bedtime buckets would lie stinking in the bedrooms. Cooking fat was left in the pan for days, the mice tracks tracing a path across it. As often as he could, Joe would stay at his grandparents, as he could not bear to live in such filth. His dad never worked. He lived on benefits and would go every day to the betting office to gamble away the valuable food money on horses. He would sometimes bring home bacon on payment day, cooking it and eating the lean whilst leaving the fat for the kids. Joe was one of eight children, the second oldest of six brothers along with his two sisters, who all co–existed in a three bedroom house on a council estate, fighting for bed space in the two small bedrooms which they shared.

Joe's clothes were threadbare and hole–ridden and never clean. He would put cardboard in his shoes to stop the dirt and wet from getting in through the holes. He would often be sent home from school because he was filthy and had not been washed. His mother would blame him for her shame and hit him with a brush. One morning before school he called for his friend, who was eating cereal. Joe had never seen cereal, never had breakfast. He would eat one meal every day at school, receiving free school dinners as the family was poor, even during the school holidays when the school would open the kitchens for the poor children at lunchtime. He would eat anything that he could find to sustain himself — apples stolen from the orchard, vegetables from gardens and farmers fields which he would steal and eat raw. Stealing was not a choice but a survival strategy.

By the age of twelve he hated school and knew that he would not survive it for another four years. He would much rather have been outside digging a hole than learning in class. Even though he was clever, from the age of twelve he would often miss school, going in to get his mark and then leaving with his friends. Although a well-built youth he hated bullies and, although scared of no-one, he was never a fighter. His entertainments were more about money, challenging friends to race round the estate and whoever won got the pot.

He began to earn his keep at the age of eight, delivering firewood for his uncle and granddad, being rewarded with a penny each Saturday for his work. At the age of thirteen he began working for a local farmer delivering milk and cream and because he drank so much milk and cream he put on two stone. By the time that he reached the age of fourteen he realised that a quick way to earn money would be to become a burglar.

His very first burglary was from the cricket club. He stole the whole stock of cigarettes which his dad took from him. The next development on his career path was to get a gang together to burgle a house. Their stash was a few thousand pounds and Joe put the whole lot in his pockets until they divided it up. They went to Blackpool on the run, but after they had slept on the beach the police caught up with them and they were arrested. Fifteen young men were in court and only Joe was found guilty! He was sentenced to go to the detention centre, but was only there for three months as his dad raised an appeal, claiming that it was unjust for only one of fifteen to be penalised. Joe then teamed up with a friend of his brother who was twenty-three years old and was a car burglar. Joe carried on burgling with him and, again, they were arrested. His brother's friend convinced Joe to plead guilty as he was underage, which Joe did, and this gained him another three months in Borstal.

Joe did not learn from his mistakes and, when he was released, he again teamed up with the same man. Joe was caught with fifty pounds worth of lead and was again sentenced to Borstal. The time detained in Borstal didn't bother Joe for there at least he was fed, clean and warm.

I remember a story that he liked to tell. He was burgling a house in the dark, which was usually the case, but there was something different about the room in which he found himself. He could hear something on chains in the corner running towards him then stopping dead, but there was no sound, no growl. He had no idea what this could be and, although he was never fearful, something about the presence in that room scared him so much that he forgot about the burgling and jumped back out of the window. He still wondered about what was chained in the corner until he died.

During this period Joe held down several jobs — a labourer in a foundry, a stonemason, a steeplejack — but his jobs were short-lived, not because he wasn't prepared to work hard, but he was easily bored.

He was not a violent man. He described himself as being like a cat. He was fast and afraid of nothing. He was a loner, plying his trade in the early hours of the morning. He only ever took cash, nothing else, and never hurt anyone. He didn't squander his ill-gotten gains on gambling, drugs and alcohol like most of the other young men; he would buy cows so that they could make money for him. He knew what to look for in a good cow, maybe from being around them when he was delivering for the farmer, and two friends let him keep them on their farms.

Another arrest led to another sentence, a week before his twenty-first birthday, after he agreed to burgle some silver from a house for someone else. He only took the job because times were hard. The police missed him and he went on the run for six months, but they never gave up their search and eventually he was caught and sent to prison.

His girlfriend at the time visited him every day. Joe was very much in love with her, his first love, and they had a daughter together. They were married whilst Joe was still in prison and, although not an ideal situation, he was content that they could start a new life when he was released. Unfortunately, things didn't quite work out as planned and they went their separate ways.

Prison was not a good place to be but it did teach Joe something. He was in jail for years for stealing small bits of cash that never amounted to anything. There was a man in jail with him who had embezzled hundreds of thousands of pounds and he was only in for six months. Joe sat and considered the rich of this world: boxers, racing drivers, business men. There are so many boxers who have tried and failed to make it big, the same with racing drivers. However, there are millions of business men and thousands of those have had great success one way or another. So he surmised from this small acorn of understanding that this was his best option; to become a business man. He decided there and then that he would use the system to stay on the right side of the law. He was confident that he could turn his life around and make the millions that he had always dreamed of because in reality the business man in jail with him was no better or cleverer than himself.

Joe was finally released at the age of twenty–two. He caught the bus home and was so happy to find his dog, which he loved, waiting at the bus stop for him. He lived with his mother for a while, back in his old neighbourhood, and soon returned to his old trade. But this time he had a purpose because he was trying to raise money to buy a demolition job with his friend. He had to raise one thousand pounds for his share of the job. He raised the money and had twenty men working for him on it. It took three months to complete and he never made a penny, breaking even from the lead and the timber which he sold. He went into partnership with his friend, but this was short–lived as they disagreed on how things should be done. Joe gained another demolition job by himself in Keighley. He recalled how he nearly killed himself on that job. He cut a steel girder and intended to jump out of the way of its fall, but the girder fell quicker than he had anticipated. Luckily it wedged between two walls, otherwise his journey to his millions might have ended abruptly that day.

He had various business partners as time went by, but he realised some thirty years ago that the only way in which he would succeed was if he worked alone, which is what he did. I met him shortly afterwards when he had just set up his demolition company and had one machine, one car and one house, all on finance or mortgaged.

I met Joe on a blind date set up by one of my friends when I was eighteen and Joe was thirty–three. When Joe first saw me he thought that I looked like trouble, or so he said, and didn't think that he had much chance with me. To me he just seemed uninterested. As the evening drew to a close, a group of us went back to Joe's house. Things improved and Joe and I sat on the sofa chatting, ignoring the drunken antics of the others in the sauna and Jacuzzi. I still remember his–ice blue trousers with brown socks and white shoes — luckily it didn't put me off! He playfully tried to carry me to the bedroom and, as I resisted, he accidentally ripped my dress.

The following day I was helping out in a sports shop where I used to be the manageress before I started modelling and who should walk in but Joe. He gave me one hundred pounds, a lot of money in those days, to buy myself a new dress to replace the one that he had ripped.

And that was that. We quickly became a couple and spent much time playing and partying, the same as anyone in a new relationship.

We married after a short while and I gave birth to our daughter, Jenna, when I was twenty years old. Jenna was the apple of our eyes, but we planned another child and Jordan, our son, was born on Joe's fortieth birthday. We now had a large family as Joe already had three children from a previous marriage who visited every weekend, so life was pretty busy. It was a hard struggle to begin with and Joe was not the easiest person to live with. I never asked about his business affairs — I didn't need to know — as long as he looked after our children and me then I was happy. I loved him so very much and he was my idol — he was like a father–figure and very protective. He was such a hard–working man, often having to work away from home for weeks at a time.

Demolition was Joe's passion and it was eventually in demolition that Joe made his millions. He tried his luck in other businesses: a bike supermarket, a restaurant and wine bar, a club and various properties. But it was in demolition that his common sense and ability to learn quickly made him an expert. Before he died he had achieved his dream of becoming a millionaire; he bought his dream house (a farm with one hundred and ten acres), his dream boat (a seventy–five foot motor yacht) and various commercial properties. He travelled the world in luxury and owned two aeroplanes during his lifetime. He was a self–made man who enjoyed life to the full. His motto in life was always to spend half and save half and that never really changed. He was very proud of his achievements and would often sit looking at one of his properties or driving around them, proud that he had made so much for himself and his family from nothing by his hard work and determination, proud of the fruits of his labour and love.

Joe was just a man like any other. His beginnings were lowly and, even though he had strong loyalties and survival instincts, he was drawn to a life away from the straight and narrow. There weren't exactly many job opportunities open for people born into those circumstances so this isn't as strange as it sounds. I am not trying to justify his actions in any way. This was a young man raised in poverty with very little hope of ever leaving it. This was my husband, warts and all, and I loved him dearly.

He was no philosopher or man of learning, but his words of wisdom were that life is just a blink of the eye lid, and that before you know it your life will be over so enjoy it while you can. He would say that he had nothing to come back for because he had done it all. His favourite sayings were that you can't live forever and it's only money! You can't take it with you!

He was something of a joker though. He once sold a 500 BSA motorbike for five pounds. The man could not pay Joe all at once, so Joe said that he could pay him in weekly instalments. The man was tinkering with the bike one day when a man passed by and shouted 'hey, that's my bike', and took the bike back. The buyer rang Joe, cursing that the bike hadn't been his to sell, to which Joe answered 'I never said it was!' Sounds like Joe.

As I said at the beginning, Joe was just a man trying to make his way in the world in the best way that he could. From a start in life on the wrong side of the law, he bettered himself and grew to be a loyal man who loved his family and the people close to him, even though he showed it by deeds rather than words and sentiment. We shared a wonderful life of good times and bad like every marriage, times of plenty and times of hardship, but through it all he said that I had made him the happiest man ever and that he adored me for being such a good mother. He also told me that he loved me more than anything, words that I'll treasure forever.

Photographs

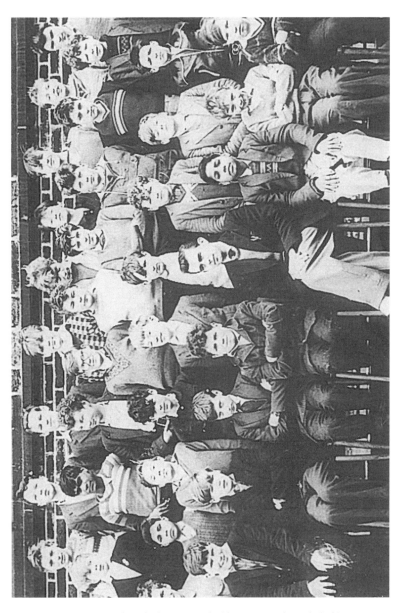

Joe school photograph (front row fourth left)

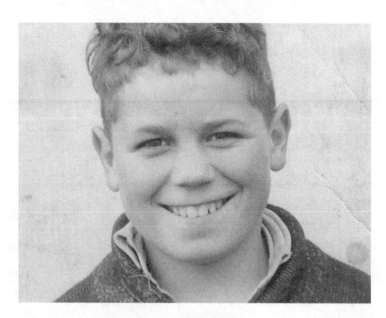

Young Joe

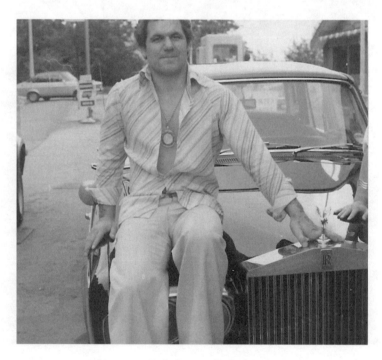

Joe's first Rolls Royce

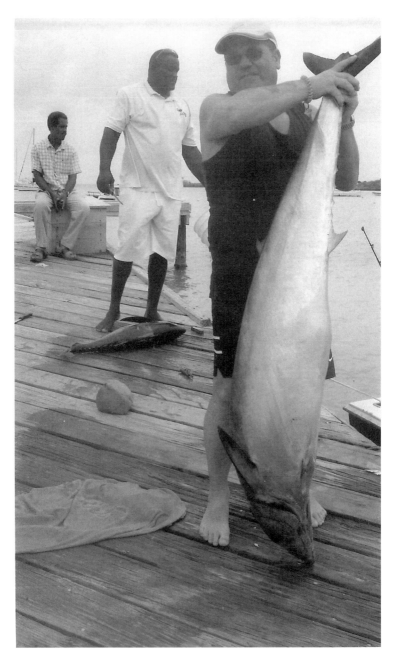

Joe and the whale

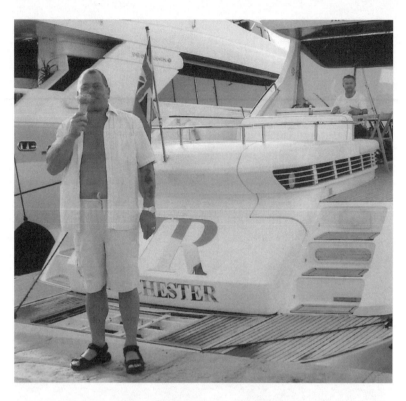

Joe in front of his boat

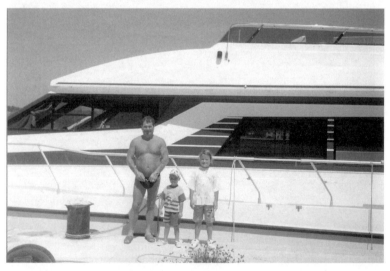

Joe, Jenna and Jordan in front of boat

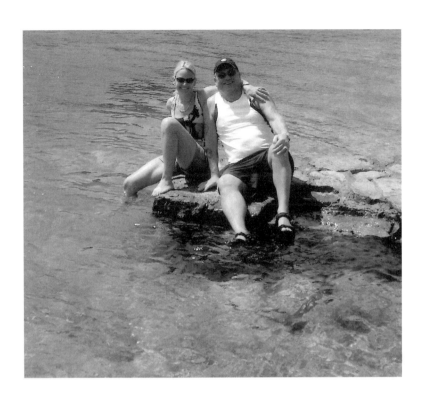

Julie and Joe in Croatia 2008

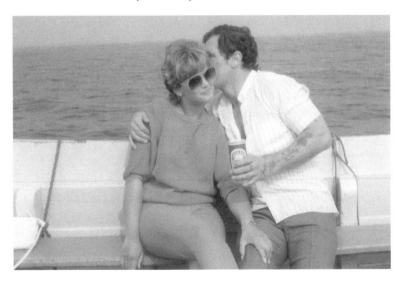

Julie and Joe the early days

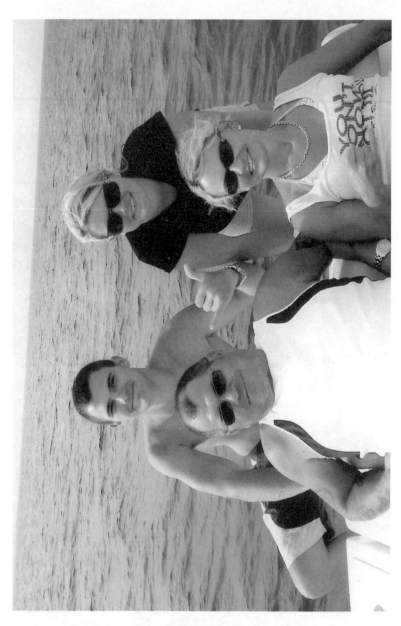

Joe, Julie, Jenna and Jordan 2006

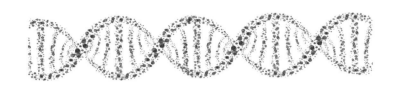

3 — The Diagnosis

Our journey began on the 18th November 2004.

I was recovering in hospital, having just undergone an operation to remove a breast lump. Being ever the optimist I hadn't even given a thought as to whether it might be cancer — or so I told myself — but I was still relieved to have it out of my body. It was Joe's birthday so I was focused on being out of bed in time to celebrate with him, and also with our son who shared the same birthday. Being in bed was something of a rare treat, time to think for a change as my life was so full and busy. The fact that Joe was downstairs having a consultation for the results of a biopsy on his prostate was momentarily forgotten, insignificant anyway since I was sure that it would be clear.

Joe burst into the room, large as life as always. No preamble, no niceties, he simply blurted out 'I've got cancer'. I struggled to make sense of his words through the fuzziness of the anaesthetic. Surely I had misheard. Did he say my lump was cancer? Did he say that he had cancer? The room fell silent and empty as he turned and left, telling me that he was going to get a newspaper, everything back to normal, as though my world had not just crashed down around me.

We had begun to suspect earlier during the year that there might be a problem, but didn't quite know what, following a facelift operation which Joe had. He had been placed on a drip post–operatively to replenish fluids and blood lost during the operation. (Fluids also need replacing due to fasting and poor intake prior to operation in many cases. Drips can also provide nutrition, **electrolytes,** glucose and water to help the patient to recover after the operation until they are back to eating normally and fully recovered after the anaesthetic. The amount of fluid given is always carefully administered so as not to give too much or too little as this can be dangerous).

During Joe's recovery it became apparent that he needed to

urinate more frequently than normal, and that it was painful when he did. The facelift had meant that Joe was under general anaesthetic for five hours. This had obviously put a tremendous strain on his immune system. As a generalisation, by the time that a cancer is found it has been manifesting for some time. It is impossible to medically prove for how long the cancer has been growing. Therefore, I can only assume that the cancer was already in the prostate and that this operation increased the symptoms significantly enough for it to become apparent that there might be cause for concern.

Also during 2004 Joe had been going for regular health checks with a private doctor. He had initially consulted him as he was concerned that his sex drive was not what it should be. Our sex life had always been very active, probably due as much to the fact that I was fifteen years younger than Joe. Joe thought that testosterone tablets would do the trick, but the doctor did not want to prescribe them. They may well have solved the dysfunction, but until the root cause of the problem could be ascertained then testosterone tablets could do more harm than good. The reducing libido, coupled with a need to urinate more often, quite often painfully, led the doctor to diagnose Joe's condition as potential **prostatitis**, a condition where the prostate is enlarged, causing pain when urinating and requiring urination more frequently. Joe was given some pills to treat the prostatitis. The doctor also carried out a rectal examination so that he could feel whether the size of the prostate appeared normal. His conclusion was that there was nothing untoward. The doctor also carried out some blood tests. When the results came back they indicated that further investigation was recommended due to the **PSA** level in the blood being slightly raised. However, at that stage the doctor did not request any further tests as the PSA was within normal range at 3.47.

PSA is a protein produced by the cells of the prostate gland and is often elevated in men with prostate cancer. However, it can also be elevated in men with prostatitis. There is no evidence to suggest that men with prostatitis will go on to develop prostate cancer. The ceiling for a normal PSA reading is 4.0 which was the reason for the suggestion for further tests in Joe's case, because although in the normal range it was high and when taking the other symptoms into consideration it could potentially be an indication of cancer. This is not an exact science — it is possible for men with higher PSA readings than 4.0 not to have prostate cancer and for men with lower readings than 4.0 to have prostate cancer. It is merely an indicator and should be considered along with other factors. (There is a new gene-based urine test out now called **PCA3**. This is not a replacement for the normal PSA testing but an additional tool to help to decide whether men with a higher PSA reading might need a biopsy to rule out prostate cancer).

Joe decided to seek another opinion and see if he could obtain the testosterone tablets elsewhere. We spent quite a lot of time in Spain as we had a house there, and we therefore decided to seek the opinion of a local Spanish doctor. Joe was convinced that testosterone tablets were the answer to his lowered sex drive and other problems, but again the doctor would not give them to him. He did, however, suggest that he should have further investigations.

The pain when urinating continued to get worse. Joe would wake up several times during the night to go to the toilet. Sometimes when we were driving he would have to stop the car mid journey and relieve himself at the roadside as the pain would become so intense until he did so. Eventually Joe could stand no more and had to resign himself to the fact that he must go back to the doctor in the UK.

Back to the UK doctor who again examined the prostate. He said that it felt a little hard but not enlarged. However, he said that he would send Joe for a biopsy as a precaution. So at this point there was still no real suspicion that prostate cancer was a possibility.

That was until 18th November 2004 when Joe was told that he had prostate cancer. The doctor tried to alleviate Joe's anxiety.

'Don't worry you are not going to die of it,' he smiled.

'Oh, that's funny, my wife is upstairs and she has got cancer too,' replied Joe, joking but it had obviously crossed his mind.

When the private doctor heard that Joe had been diagnosed with prostate cancer he was distraught, especially since by the time that it was diagnosed it had already spread to his bones. He said that he did not sleep for a week after I called him to tell him the bad news. He blamed himself for mis-diagnosing Joe. He felt incompetent that his training as a GP was not geared towards specialist diagnosis and felt compelled to give up his practice. The GP sent letters out to all of his patients informing them of his resignation from private practice. His words to me were, 'as a GP I am not a specialist in any field and, because of this, mis-diagnosis can occur. For these reasons I am unhappy to continue practicing as a GP'.

Was he to blame for the late diagnosis? Who knows. Looking at the evidence and the difficulty in differentiating prostatitis from prostate cancer it could potentially be mis–diagnosed. However, Joe had been going to this doctor annually for several years for health checks and there were problems evident in the blood reports which had been received — elevated liver and kidney enzymes together with thyroid irregularities — all potential indications of an underlying problem, so maybe some alarm bells should have gone off.

GPs are the gate–keepers to the specialist and they help to guide patient's education as a disease develops. Just as a surgeon who has done one hundred operations is likely to be more successful, so too a GP, as any professional such a solicitor or an accountant, is likely to be more successful the more experienced he or she is. When one qualifies, working in teams helps to get the right mix of experience and enthusiasm for any new treatment that needs to be fully assessed before becoming routine.

Today computers facilitate the monitoring of experience. I once visited a newly qualified doctor. On her wall were a number of boxes with the heading 'breast lump'. From the boxes displayed, the doctor had to decide which one to tick. This box then led to more boxes and one box had to be ticked again. This eventually led to either a specialist appointment, a follow–up appointment, self–monitoring. A GP is not a specialist and, like any professional, some are more naturally gifted than others. Just as an accountant may know everything that there is to know about budgeting but know only what they studied in their exams about tax, they can't know everything about everything. Doctors, specialists and GPs are only human and can, therefore, sometimes get it wrong, so it is always best if unsure to get a second opinion.

To reaffirm this point, I once showed my GP a small mark on my back. I was told that I could have a life–threatening cancer and must go and have it looked at immediately. I was due to go on holiday the next day, flying from London, so I arranged to see a skin specialist there. He laughed and told me not to worry as it was definitely not cancer, suggesting that he could remove it on my return to the UK. Subsequently, on my return I met with Professor Oliver (discussed later) who suggested that, since I had two conflicting opinions, I should seek a further opinion before removal. The skin specialist in Yorkshire was mortified to hear of my worry over something which was, he confirmed, nothing whatsoever. Another mistake — or simply caution due to lack of experience in this area?

Unfortunately, when people become ill and visit the doctor, some people listen to these doctors like they are Gods (no disrespect intended) and believe every word that they say, quite rightly recognising that the doctor knows much more than they do so must be correct. Some people can be too accepting of their fate to question anything about their illness and just go along with everything which they are told. Then there are the people like me who never give up questioning until they are satisfied. Undoubtedly there are many brilliant doctors out there and some amazing specialists and professors — it is simply a matter of finding them.

I think that the word of caution here is for you to use your own judgment about what you are being told. If you are told that the PSA is toward the ceiling of normal and there is a problem with painful urination, then this should be a red flag to insist on further tests. What can be lost by doing more tests except NHS money and, although budgets and funds are important, this should be a low priority compared to saving someone's life?

Having the confidence to be insistent about your treatment can be a powerful tool in the early stages. A friend of mine has a husband with prostate cancer. She has no academic background, just the same burning desire to save her husband. He was diagnosed very early, mainly thanks to his wife. He had no other symptoms except that on just a few occasions he had felt the need to urinate more frequently than usual when he had drunk slightly more fluids. Because his wife had read a lot about prostate cancer, just from the news and so forth, she immediately demanded the relevant tests and he was diagnosed at an early stage. As I said, she has no academic background and isn't computer literate, but she researched everything that she could. Before making any decisions or being steered towards a particular path of treatment she made sure that she had all of the facts, not just the facts that the hospital was able to give her. Her husband's treatment has been on the NHS and she has given him a better quality of life by choosing wisely which treatments he will receive and by fighting for the treatments which they didn't want to give, even treatments which are available on the NHS but are not readily offered because of the cost.

The power to choose and take control is in your hands.

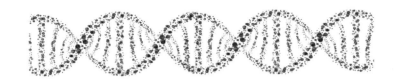

4 — First Steps

Recommended Treatments

The results of the biopsy showed cancerous **tumours** in every one of the **core** samples extracted. The tumour had a **Gleason score** of seven. Without going into too much detail, the Gleason score is a grading system used by pathologists to indicate how aggressive the cancer is. The higher the Gleason score the more aggressive is the cancer. Scores of two to four indicate a cancer which is low on the aggression scale, scores of five and six are mildly aggressive. A score of seven indicates that the cancer is moderately aggressive. Scores between eight and ten mean that the cancer is very aggressive. Consequently Joe's cancer was quite an aggressive prostate cancer. There was no indication of perineural invasion (cancer spreading to the nerve surrounding the tissue) or lymphovascular invasion (spreading to the blood vessels) identified.

There are various methods of treatment available for prostate cancer and various combinations of treatment which are dependent upon the state of the prostate and the stage of the cancer at the time of diagnosis. It is extremely important to initially research all of the available options and treatments. It is then vitally important to obtain a firm understanding of whether the cancer is low, medium or high risk so that the relevant options can be better assessed for your individual stage of illness. High risk means that there is a high probability of a secondary cancer developing or already being present. Each individual has different priorities and different factors affecting their decision on which treatment route to follow dependent on such issues as age, other health problems, side–effects from treatments and family commitments and concerns. Also, if you are in doubt about the treatment being offered or your understanding of the treatment, then don't be afraid to request a second opinion, even if it is just a matter of wanting to increase certainty about the options available — your doctor will want to be sure that you understand your options and diagnosis so this shouldn't be a problem. Insist on scans whenever possible to rule out **metastatic** disease. Supposition is all very well, but it doesn't save lives when too late it comes to light that the supposition was flawed. Obviously the sooner that metastatic disease is diagnosed the better.

Here are brief explanations of the recommended available treatments which are generally offered — this list is not exhaustive as new treatments become available every day.

DRE Tests – Digital Rectal Exam

The doctor inserts a gloved and lubricated finger into the rectum to identify any abnormalities with the shape or texture of the prostate. The prostate can also be massaged prior to performance of the PCA3 test. This is a very basic first stage test.

PSA Tests

This is a simple blood test which measures how much PSA (Prostate–Specific Antigen) is in the body as elevated levels could indicate prostate cancer, but it could also indicate prostatitis or enlarged prostate. Also, men with cancer may not show elevated PSA levels. Further tests should be performed in conjunction with this test. A level of below 4 has generally been accepted as normal. However, PSA levels in younger men are lower so the ceiling for results should be lowered in such cases.

PCA3 Tests

This is a new test based on DNA technology which provides a more efficient means of detecting prostate cancer than the standard PSA test and helps to discriminate between high and low–risk prostate cancer. This new urine test can help to avoid the need for prostate biopsies.

Active Surveillance

The cancer is closely monitored with the aid of PSA tests, DRE tests, PCA3 tests and routine biopsies at set times. It is because prostate cancer surgery has to be so extensive and risks serious complications that, if the initial diagnostic tests suggest a low level of malignancy, such patients may undergo a period of 'watch and wait' which involves no specific, immediate treatment.

This approach is generally used on younger patients as it is likely that they have more to gain from tolerating the side–effects of treatment. At any time a decision can be taken to begin treatment. This was not an option for Joe.

Radical Prostatectomy

This involves the surgical removal of the prostate gland. For patients with early stage, organ–confined prostate cancer, a nerve–sparing **prostatectomy** is a more likely option. With nerve–sparing prostatectomy the risks of erectile dysfunction and incontinence are lowered, these being the two major risk factors. If the cancer cells have started to spread outside of the prostate, typically in Joe's case, nerve–sparing prostatectomy is more difficult as more tissue needs to be removed to try to ensure that all of the cancer is captured.

Radiotherapy for Prostate Cancer

There are two ways of giving radiotherapy for prostate cancer; one uses an external beam and the other is internal and is called **Brachytherapy.** This internal treatment is becoming more popular as it is a fairly simple and successful treatment with very little radiation reaching adjacent normal organs. However, it may not always be effective on its own and may also need external radiotherapy alongside it. We were not offered this treatment as Joe's cancer was too advanced.

When I studied the possible side–effects of external beam radiotherapy, which Joe was offered as an alternative to radical prostatectomy, the side–effects and risks seemed to be worse than with the prostatectomy. The short–term side–effects can be bladder inflammation, diarrhoea, sore skin in the treatment area and loss of pubic hair, whilst the long–term side–effects can be inflammation to the rectum, frequent or loose bowel movements, difficulty in passing urine due to the narrowing of the pipe between the bladder and the penis and also erectile dysfunction. When considering this now, had we opted for the radiotherapy, things could have turned out much worse as we would not have known the extent to which the cancer had already spread and been able to take action until it was probably much too late, action which we were able to take following radical prostatectomy.

Hormone Therapy Treatment

This standalone treatment is an option for men who are not well enough for surgery or radiotherapy, or for those whose cancer has already spread to the bones, like Joe. Hormone therapy treats prostate cancer by various methods, but all **hormone therapy treatments** have the same aim — to prevent testosterone from feeding the cancer cells as without it the cancer cells will grow more slowly and this will keep the cancer cells under control for many months to many years depending on the severity of the cancer. But it will not kill the cancer cells. Hormone therapy can be used pretty much in conjunction with most other treatments. One medical professional recommended this as a standalone treatment without surgery for Joe, but we decided to opt for surgery thinking that this would be a 'quick fix' as we didn't believe that the cancer had spread.

HIFU Prostate Treatment

HIFU (High Intensity Frequency Ultrasound) is a new treatment and was not available to us at the time. A beam produces high frequency sound waves directing the beam to the tumour site. It works by heating and destroying cancer cells but not harming healthy tissue. As a result it can be focused on only the area in the prostate that has cancer and hence produce less damage than full surgery in early cases.

It is a simple procedure taking approximately four hours under general anaesthetic and patients are usually able to return home the same day. Incontinence and impotency are very low following HIFU compared with other treatments. As long term follow-up data is still not available for ten to fifteen years after diagnosis it is still experimental for early stage prostate cancer patients and those with a short life expectancy due to other conditions. Even if this treatment had been available at the time it would not have been an option for Joe as his cancer was too advanced at the time of diagnosis.

Cryosurgery for Prostate Cancer

This is another treatment which was not available at the time. This treatment is used to treat certain cancers and certain pre-cancerous conditions. The cancer cells are destroyed by freezing them. It is sometimes used for early stage prostate cancer which is confined to the prostate gland. However, it is less established than standard treatments and long-term outcomes are not yet known, though the results are possibly slightly better than HIFU due to frozen tissue possibly acting as a better tumour vaccine than heated tissue. However, longer follow-up will be required before this can be fully established.

Abiraterone Treatment for Late Stage Cancer

This drug, first discovered in this country some time ago but not developed because its full mechanism of action had not been worked out, became available half-way through Joe's treatment. I tried so hard to get my hands on this new drug. Following much research I was convinced that it would work for Joe and I was extremely hopeful that we could get another year of life at least. I tried every avenue to obtain this drug. Professor Oliver kindly wrote to the hospital which was performing the trials recommending Joe for this treatment. I wrote begging letters myself and even offered donations for Joe to be on one of the trials but they would not take him because he had already had multiple other treatments and was ineligible for the rather restrictive trials that had to be completed before it could be licenced. I was subsequently with Professor Oliver and he told me that other patients of his at an earlier stage of their disease had been accepted for **abiraterone**. Frustrating doesn't even begin to cover it. It became available under licence in September 2011 — eight months too late.

It would seem that this is a good option for men with late stage cancer who have failed all other treatments. It blocks an enzyme that is critical in the production of sex hormones, **androgens** and oestrogen. Blocking this enzyme prevents androgens from being made in the testes and other tissues in the body. It is providing extended life for people like Joe.

Joe's Options

In Joe's case a specialist surgeon in Yorkshire advised that Joe could choose between surgery to remove the prostate or external beam radiotherapy. The specialist advised that he would recommend the surgery and could operate on the 5th January 2005. Joe was told that there could be problems of erectile dysfunction and incontinence with both methods, but that if surgery was chosen he would try to spare the nerves during the surgery to prevent this. We later found out that in America they can actually replace the nerve at the same time as the operation to remove the prostate to prevent potential nerve damage. We also learnt later, after the operation, that there are some very good specialist surgeons in London with track record success, specialising in sparing the nerves during prostatectomy.

Chemotherapy was not an option at this stage as chemotherapy is not usually a first line treatment for prostate cancer as it cannot kill it — it can only prolong life. Joe did ultimately have chemotherapy during the last year or so of his life, but this was only after all other options had been exhausted. I won't dwell on chemotherapy — there are many books in circulation on this subject already.

The decision was, therefore, between surgery and external beam radiotherapy. I researched the possible side–effects of both treatments and Joe and I discussed the options together. We believed that the risks of impotence and incontinence were higher with radiotherapy. They are a known side–effect with radiotherapy, almost a given, but with surgery they could potentially be avoided. At this point Joe did not accept that the cancer was that bad, and so his main concern was losing his manhood which he feared would happen with the radical prostatectomy. But something was telling me that the prostatectomy was what he had to have. My major concern was that to leave something so cancerous in the body could only mean that it would spread further.

Moss Reports

www.cancerdecisions.com

Cancer Decisions has many ways in which it provides up–to–date information on cancer treatments. This site offers individual Moss Reports on specific types of cancers. The reports can be browsed from an online menu and then the specific report downloaded. Their monthly electronic newsletter, ADVANCES in Cancer Treatment, is written by the well–known science writer, Ralph W. Moss, PhD. Phone consultations are available to those who purchase a Moss Report on their type of cancer. Their Professional Associate program offers patients information on healthcare providers in their local area.

The site also offers many videos about their programs, products and a video blog. The Cancer Decisions Newsletter Archives contain ten years of weekly newsletters about news on the treatment of cancer. Books and visualisation audios are also available.

Unfortunately, I did not come across this site until the sixth year of Joe's cancer. By this time we had already tried many treatments and so the advice which we received was of limited value, but for someone just beginning their research the reports and advice would be invaluable, especially since purchasing the report gives access to someone on the end of a telephone line.

The reports are extensive and may seem quite daunting at first sight as they are about four hundred pages long, but if you sift through to the information which is pertinent to your case then they are very worthwhile.

Included with kind permission from Cancer Decisions

First Meeting with the Specialist Oncologist

I researched on the internet for hours, determined to be sure of my facts. We also decided to go for a second opinion about our choices from one of the top professors in prostate cancer, Professor Jones (an alias), an expert in his field, who was based in London; he is also a top surgeon and has written many books on prostate cancer. We arrived a day before our appointment so that Joe could have a bone scan. Professor Jones examined Joe and said that the prostate felt enlarged. He said that he could operate, but that it might not be so straightforward considering how enlarged the prostate felt. When he reviewed the bone scans he looked a little unsure. He advised that he would like to do some black and white, straightforward X–rays of the bones to rule out what could be signs of metastatic disease. But he said that there shouldn't be a problem — he just wanted to be sure of the exact situation.

Once the X–rays had been done we were allowed to go. Professor Jones advised that he would know more once the radiologist had assessed the X–rays, but he expected that everything would be fine. He asked that we stay around London until he had the results just in case Joe needed to have another scan the following day. He would call us when the radiologist had reported his findings to him.

We waited for the phone call in a hotel near the train station. Although neither of us had much of an appetite we went for something to eat and a bottle of wine. The phone rang. It was Professor Jones. He needed us to return to the hospital the following morning for another consultation, not for Joe to have another scan.

His tone strange, he told us to go and book into the best hotel in London and have the time of our lives! Now we were worried. There must be something seriously wrong.

We did not go to the most expensive hotel — what was there to celebrate? And we didn't want to tempt fate by guessing and commiserating. We went to one of our usual hotels and drank copious amounts of red wine. I think we actually fell asleep holding the glasses and woke up the following day surrounded by empty bottles! Oblivion is sometimes good.

Back at the hospital we were met by Professor Jones' assistant who called us in for the meeting. He was very sympathetic but that didn't change the words which he conveyed. He told us that he had bad news, that the cancer had spread to the bones and there was no point in operating. He advised that he would like to begin hormone therapy treatment straight away to prevent the cancer from spreading further. This was to be in the form of an injection which had to be injected into Joe's stomach. Joe asked how long he had left to live. We were told that the prognosis was anywhere between two and five years. It was known for one in ten 'lucky' people to have up to ten years. When later I looked at the statistics they confirmed that only a third of late–stage diagnosis patients would survive for five years and there was no data that I could find beyond five years.

The assistant explained that the hormone therapy would be administered every three months and would usually be effective for about two years, after which time the cancer would become resistant to it. After this there were no other treatments that were effective against advanced prostate cancer, not even chemotherapy. So he was telling us that Joe had two years. I began to cry, not that it would do any good, but ….. there were no words — what was there to say?

The assistant then administered the **goserelin** injection, the hormone therapy, into Joe's stomach. We were told that we could come back for the next injection in three months time or have it done by our local doctor. Joe had also already been taking **bicalutamide**, which had been prescribed by the surgeon in Yorkshire to help reduce the risks of localised spreading of the cancer around the prostate which could be missed and therefore not removed during the surgery (margin positivity), planned for January 2005.

Conflicting Opinions

We took the train home, hardly speaking during the whole journey. We were devastated. I can remember the feeling as if it was yesterday — our life was shattered. Our dreams, our hopes, our future — what future? What did the future now hold? Only uncertainty, misery, pain, death. These things happen every day, but to other people. You never believe that one day it will be you who is told that you will die. Of course we will all die, but as long as you don't know when, each day you can believe that it will not be today. Once you have been told that you have terminal cancer, then each day you start to believe that it could be your last.

I contacted the specialist in Yorkshire and updated him with the findings from the specialist in London, advising him that, judging by the results of the bone scans, it appeared that the cancer had already spread and that there would be no point in operating. The Yorkshire specialist was shocked and in disbelief. He suggested that Joe have an MRI scan as he had previously had patients denied curative surgery because some bone scan readings turned out to be false positives due to arthritis and there was no spread to the bones. The MRI scan was quickly organized and, once the results were available, I had a meeting with the radiologist who explained the films to me. He reported that there were several **lesions** on the spine but he was of the opinion that these were degenerative disease in keeping with Joe's extensive manual labour during his youth and he did not suspect these lesions to be metastatic. Both the radiologist and the surgeon were extremely convincing that this was definitely not metastatic disease. However, in London they were quite adamant, and as it turned out rightly so, that Joe did indeed have quite extensive metastatic disease despite his relatively low PSA.

These two conflicting opinions were being held by two highly trained teams of experts in their field. We could not understand how this could happen, believing that medicine was a more exact science. We would never have anticipated that we would be in a position where we were expected to make decisions when we could not possibly know the correct information, because one team was wrong and we knew not which one. We did not want to believe the worst, that the cancer had already spread. We had to take some action and desperately wanted to believe the Yorkshire specialists when they told us that the cancer had not spread, so we therefore decided that it would be best for Joe to have the operation, as something so cancerous was surely better out than in, and if it hadn't spread then removing it was the only way to stop it spreading. We knew that there were going to be risks with the operation but we thought that we would take a gamble. We hoped that Joe would be lucky and that the nerves would be spared, and that Joe would not have any problems with erectile dysfunction or incontinence. The statistics showed that nerve damage and erectile dysfunction were not high risk side–effects. The surgeon reassured us that radical prostatectomy was the best thing to do as, in this situation, there is some evidence that if there is more cancer in the primary than outside then the growth may be slowed.

A Holiday Before Battle

We had a Christmas holiday booked to Phuket, Thailand. There was nothing that we could do until Joe had his operation, so we decided to go and Joe would have the operation when we got back. We were trying to enjoy the time and relax so that Joe would be rested for when his trials began. To be honest, we were trying not to think that this could be our last holiday together. Little did we know that we were almost right in our fears, but for a very different reason!

We were lying in bed, having spent a late night in the underground nightclub.

'Are you shaking the bed? What are you doing?' he moaned.

'Nothing, it's not me.' Then the whole floor began moving from side to side and creaking eerily. The wardrobes were rattling.

'It's an earthquake!' Joe cried. 'Quick, let's get out!' We banged on the adjoining room where Jenna, our daughter, and Jordan, our son, were sleeping and shouted, 'get out, it's an earthquake!'

Jenna, who had a hangover from the night before, didn't want to move and told us to leave her. Even though I screamed repeatedly that I wasn't joking, it was an earthquake, she wouldn't budge. Eventually we forced her out of the bed. We ran downstairs to find people rushing around in pyjamas, panicked and scared. The hotel stood its ground and we were unharmed, just shaken — literally! We ate breakfast early. We were told that the earthquake had hit many other parts of the globe also. After breakfast things settled down a little and Joe wanted to go to the main Phuket town, the events of the early morning wake–up already forgotten. I was not keen on the idea as the beach there was not good — there were many old men there with young Thai women — so I didn't feel comfortable. Nor did I want to go to the shops — the weather was too nice — so I decided to stay at our hotel. Joe and Jordan went off to Phuket town to window shop. Joe warned that we should take care as there may be aftershocks. He really wanted us to go with him, maybe because he'd feel better just in case, knowing where we were and that we were safe. Thank goodness that we did not.

The beach was protected by a low wall with steps leading up to a long grass verge. Jenna and I settled down on the grass to sunbathe, not quite at ease remembering Joe's warning. A sense of foreboding fell upon me — maybe I subconsciously heard the pandemonium — and I stood, looking towards the sea. What I saw froze me with fear. The sea was rushing up over the beach, boats swirling like flotsam and washing up towards the beach wall. There were no sunbeds or umbrellas to be seen — they had all been washed away. The ladies working on the beach ran screaming as the water swept around them and washed all of their things away. Then, as fast as the sea had rampaged across the beach, it pulled itself away completely, taking everything in its path with it. Bewilderment took over any common sense and fear as everyone stood hypnotised. Then I saw it on the horizon, the most enormous wave. I yelled to Jenna to run. Everyone was running, knocking each other out of the way. We ran through the hotel and hijacked a taxi with another lady who had two small children. We screamed for him to drive to the highest point. The taxi driver reassured us that he knew where the highest point was. He drove as fast as the fleeing crowds would allow. We asked the taxi driver if this had happened before and he told us that he had never seen anything like it.

We found ourselves atop a high mountain in our bikinis. The sun was scorching hot, we had no money, no mobile phone, nothing. We'd left everything on the sun loungers, forgotten in the panic to escape the surging wall of water. The lady with the two children took shelter in a local's shack and they made food and drinks for her and the children. Her husband was out fishing. I remember thinking that it would have been a different story for us if this had happened the night before when we had been in the underground nightclub in the hotel.

Once the panic had died down and the waters had stopped rising our thoughts turned to Joe and Jordan. There was a bar a short way down the hillside and we decided to climb down to find out if there was a telephone to call them. Panic stirred as I feared what might have happened to my husband and my son. When we arrived at the bar we were hit by the reality of the extent of the tsunami. We hadn't realised how terrible it was and were unable to comprehend the devastation which surrounded us. The worst hit area was the main Phuket beach where we should have been, where Joe and Jordan were. Desperately I repeatedly tried to call Joe from the telephone in the bar. Finally I reached him. Thank the Lord that they were safe. They had seen people running and had followed. Glass windows had been smashing around them and they had needed to climb over walls to escape. Thank goodness that Joe had been in training pre–operation to get himself fit and healthy. He said that he had found our car and that it was underwater but he had managed to bucket the water out of the car and amazingly it started. He drove to find us on the mountain side. Finally we were all together. The sea was extremely violent for the rest of the day and there were warnings of more tsunamis, but even stronger. These warnings went on all day through loudspeakers, delivered from cars driving round the parts of the town which were not too deep with water, telling us to stay on the mountain and away from the beaches.

We stayed up on the mountain until early evening as we had been advised. We lodged the car behind a tree in case another tsunami came. In the early evening we went back to the hotel where they warned of another tsunami through the night. Many people made their way to the airport, desperate for flights home. The poor lady with the two children was worried all day long. Her husband never called. She feared the worst. Eventually her husband rang and couldn't understand why she was so upset. He knew nothing of the tsunami. He had been oblivious and totally unaffected out at sea. We offered the lady a lift with us but she decided to stay in the shack overnight. Her husband did not even go to find her. He said that he would see her in the morning. How strange people are. I was happy that I had Joe who had been desperate to get to us.

Our hotel was closed down so we collected our belongings and we were moved to another hotel on a hillside. The new hotel was infested with giant ants, probably also having fled up the hill to escape from the water. They climbed up the mosquito nets around the beds and dropped onto them. At first they only seemed to be in the children's bedroom, but then they explored and were in mine also. Joe snored through everything, unaffected as usual. Needless to say the rest of us did not get much sleep. The following day we moved out to another hotel on the south of the island where fortunately there were rooms available. After the horrors of the previous few days it was paradise. We enjoyed the rest of the holiday as much as we could. Poor Joe must have felt that someone was definitely trying to get him one way or the other! But we were all safe.

Had we gone with Joe to Phuket town we could all have been in the sea or on the beach and not here to tell this story. We all know about the devastation of the tsunami. In a way, it put the cancer into perspective. Joe may not have had forever to live, but life can be taken at any time from any of us, and that day it could have been taken from all of us, not just Joe. Life is for living and every day could be your last whether you have cancer or not which, if you think about it, puts a whole new perspective on the way that you live your life.

The Prostatectomy

We arrived back in England on the 3rd January and Joe had his operation on the 5th January. I was with Joe as they took him down for the operation and waited for him to come back, nervous to ask what they had found. All went well with the operation, but the surgeon was unsure as to whether he had spared the nerves which was not good. Ninety per cent of the prostate gland was involved and, coupled with the Gleason score of seven, was not a good sign. Fortunately there was no spread to any of the lymph nodes which were analysed. However, after a short time the PSA started to rise again. The surgeon suggested radiotherapy but Joe would not even consider it — he had made his choice to have the operation instead of the radiotherapy and had no intention of having to have both as this would certainly take away his manhood. The surgeon advised that some cells had potentially escaped and the radiotherapy was a kind of mopping up procedure. I felt a sliver of fear slide down my back on hearing this as I had thought that once the operation was done and the tumour removed it would be plain sailing. Even though the surgeon strongly recommended the radiotherapy, Joe still refused.

After a short while it became clear that Joe's manhood had disappeared and his little friend no longer wanted to play. Joe was deeply upset as this was a major part of our married life together. He was told that it could take six to twelve months for his manhood to come back, for the nerves to repair. Sadly this never happened. However, the surgeon suggested that with the use of **viagra** and an injection of **alprostadil**, a good erection could be achieved. He wasn't kidding. One night whilst away on a trip we couldn't sleep and we were 'busy' all night. It was great to enjoy our marriage properly again. I won't go into further details, but our sex life was better than ever. Sadly this did not last long term, and after about three years the injection stopped working. But at least Joe was able to feel how he wanted to feel for a few years longer and it helped him to feel that his quality of life due to the cancer was not impaired.

This was just one of the complications with the operation. At the time you convince yourself that everything will be fine and that the healing process will be everything that it should be. Positive thinking. The other complication was the scar tissue build–up in the urinary tubes from where the prostate was removed. The scar tissue problem constantly returned and poor Joe had to be rushed into hospital to have the tube opened again and again and the scar tissue removed. Often without warning he would not be able to urinate and had to go straight to the hospital. This happened about eight times. Once it happened whilst we were in Spain which was very distressing for Joe. It is fortunate that I speak Spanish as no–one could speak English. Eventually they managed to release the urine with a catheter. We flew back to England and Joe underwent yet another operation to deal with the build–up. The staff at the clinic in Yorkshire came to know Joe very well as he turned up many times with this problem.

Following the many recurrences of this problem it was recommended that Joe use a catheter on a daily basis to prevent further build–up of the scar tissue, which he did. Had this been suggested earlier then it would have prevented the need for so many distressing minor operations to be performed to relieve the problem. Even with the catheter it was forever Joe's fear when travelling that he would have trouble urinating, so for many years he was extremely vigilant about ensuring that the catheter went wherever he went.

The difficult thing to deal with was that we had not been made aware of this possible side–effect before the operation. Not that it would have made much difference as the operation had been seen to be the best course of action, whatever the consequences, but at least we would have been prepared. Having all of the facts was a constant difficulty and the lack of information regarding possible problems was recurrent.

The Robbery

The scar build–up problem happened again late at night whilst I away was skiing in Spain with my son, so Joe had to drive himself to the hospital, have the operation and bravely drive himself home the following morning. That same early morning, my son and I were robbed by four masked men in our home in Spain. They carried screwdrivers and held them to my throat demanding money.

I was awake in my bedroom, talking on the phone to my friend, when they broke into the house. Having heard something, I opened my bedroom door and there, stood before me, were three men in balaclavas. I screamed! One of them hit me and I fell to the bed.

'Stop! Don't hit her,' another one shouted — thank goodness! Two of the robbers jumped on me and held me down. They removed all of my jewellery, including my engagement ring — thankfully they left my wedding ring. They pointed the screwdriver to my throat.

'Where's the money? Where's the safe?' The man who had stopped them from hitting me looked at me.

'It's okay, don't worry, you have too much money,' he said quietly. At that point my son burst in. They had been pushing his head into the pillow saying, 'Police! Go to sleep'. Eventually he got to my room.

'What are they doing to you, mum?' he yelled, 'what are they doing?' They grabbed his arm to remove his watch. Jordan threw a punch at them, then quickly they punched him three times in the head and threw him on the bed. They were not going to leave without money. They asked if the jewels were real and I told them that they were. I remembered that Joe had left some money in the kitchen cupboard to pay a bill, about five thousand euros. I told them that I knew where the money was and that I would take them. Once I had shown them the money in the kitchen cupboard they were sure that we had no safe. They tied us up with electric cables and straightening irons to the bathroom radiator. My only thought was that they were going to electrocute us. Thankfully they didn't. They closed the door, stole the car, which had a tracker on, and left. They were in the house for fifty minutes, during which time the phones were ringing constantly, but none of this alarmed the robbers. My friend was still on the phone and heard everything — she had called my friend in Spain and had told her to get the police, who didn't arrive until after the robbers had left. The police knew where the car was because of the tracker and they supposedly followed the car to Grenada where the robbers had abandoned it and escaped. I think the robbers originally followed us from a restaurant in Puerto Banus where we called for dinner on our way back from skiing. It's always easy to see things differently with hindsight but, looking back, I remembered some suspicious-looking men watching me as I got into the car when we left the restaurant.

I was so unsettled after this that it was a long time before I was able to go back to the house. I never felt relaxed there again until I put alarms outside in the garden and locks on all of the interior doors. Had Joe been there I am sure that he would not have survived this ordeal. He would not have sat helplessly and watched them. So again he had evaded harm — maybe someone did like him after all. Poor Joe, after driving himself from the hospital from yet another operation, took the earliest flight possible and flew out to me. He came to support me and be by my side after my ordeal. Again it was almost as though situations were being held up before us to show that cancer isn't necessarily the worst thing in life — it's just one more thing to overcome.

So we were once again back in the UK and back to the scar tissue problem. Joe often recalled a particular visit to the hospital to have his tube opened and the surgeon used a metal rod which was forced down his penis. He said it was agony! He so regretted having the operation and said that if he had known all of the consequences of having it and been aware of the fact that the cancer had already spread to the bones then he would never have had it. He laid the blame at the door of the surgeon who had talked him into having surgery. The blame, I would say, is justified as he had misled Joe into believing that the cancer had not spread to the bones.

I did not share his feelings. I was happy that he had undergone the operation despite everything. I firmly believe that if such a cancerous prostate had been left in his body that the cancer would have spread more quickly. Of course I did not have to suffer the painful results, but that made my judgment clearer. It also proves that there is never a straightforward and right decision — you just have to weight up the pros and cons and go for it. Every choice is at best an educated guess, at worst a gamble.

Joe's PSA continued to rise; not drastically, but it should not have been rising at all following the removal of the prostate, and we were therefore unclear as to whether the cancer had indeed spread. It was recommended that Joe remain on hormone therapy, so he remained on the goserelin injection every three months.

We returned to Professor Jones for Joe to have the goserelin injection. He remained convinced that the cancer had already spread to the bone. He said that he knew a top radiologist at a hospital in Birmingham and that he would send our scans to him for a second opinion if we wished. We agreed. The specialist radiologist reaffirmed that the results indicated that it was most likely that there was **metastasis** in the bones and that hormone therapy would be the best course of action.

This was always a perplexing situation. I look back now and laugh at the controversy between the results in London and the results in Yorkshire. First Professor Jones, then the Birmingham hospital and then the London clinic, were all confident that the hotspots on the bone scans were in keeping with metastatic bone disease. However, in Yorkshire they had a different opinion. In the beginning they were of the opinion that the lesions on the bone were probably from manual labour in Joe's youth and refused to acknowledge that there was evidence of metastatic disease. Then again, when Joe had pain in one of his ribs and underwent a further bone scan and a lesion was evident, they concluded that this was likely to represent a fracture, not evidence of metastatic disease. Finally, on another bone scan, even though similar hot spots (which show up as abnormal areas on the scan) were now present on two more ribs and there was an increase in activity in the thoracic spine and the mid lumbar spine, the conclusion was that this would be compatible with degenerative change and still was not convincing evidence of metastasis. Amazing! Following this we decided to have no further care in Yorkshire and all of Joe's treatments were subsequently carried out in London.

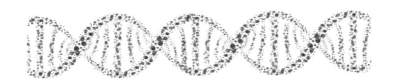

5 — Dr Hilu and Cellular Medicine Analysis

Early Days

After the prostatectomy I began to research alternative medicine treatments and cures for cancer.

Word of mouth, through a friend of a friend, led us to Dr Hilu, a cellular medicine analysis doctor in Spain. Cellular medicine analysis, also known as live blood cell analysis, nutritional microscopy or sometimes darkfield microscopy, is really quite straightforward. It involves taking a pin prick of blood from the finger and then putting it on a glass slide where it can be viewed under an extremely powerful microscope connected to a camera. As the name implies, the extracted blood cells are visible, still alive, under the microscope. The first sight of cells moving around which only seconds ago were in the body is absolutely fascinating.

A number of things can be seen by examining the blood. The condition and quality of your red blood cells have a direct impact on your present and future health, with signs of stress and disease appearing in the blood years before they manifest as a physical symptom. The aim is not to provide a diagnosis of a condition but to provide a picture of how healthy we are from the inside out based on findings in the cellular medicine analysis.

There has long been a popular saying that 'life is in the blood' and as with all life the blood is constantly changing. The red blood cells live for about one hundred to one hundred and twenty days and consequently the whole blood can change in three to four months. There is much controversy over what can be seen in the blood and there are many inexperienced people practicing blood microscopy, so beware! There are no licensing requirements to perform this analysis as a service. The main concept to understand is that from the cellular medicine analysis the general health of the patient can be seen and, above all, the general state of the immune system is revealed. The relationship between the human immune system and cancer is important to understand when assessing potential cancer treatments. This is best described by the experts: *www.cancerresearch.org/cancer-immunotherapy/what-is-cancer-immunotherapy*

Examples of the potential problems which are visible from the cellular medicine analysis are:

- Acidity in the body
- Fat content in the blood/body
- Digestive problems
- Toxicity
- Crystals
- Allergies
- Dehydration
- Deficiencies
- Circulatory dysfunctions
- Hormonal imbalances
- Oxidative stress
- Degenerative tendencies

This list is by no means exhaustive but provides an overview of the most common issues.

First Visits

We first visited Dr Hilu at his clinic in Torremolinos, close to the airport in Malaga, Spain, on 31st May 2005.

Dr Hilu is a very positive and confident figure, obviously extremely important characteristics for someone in whom you are placing your trust. There is no uncertainty in anything which he advises you and his experience means that he knows exactly down which path to lead you. Dr Hilu gave us our initial and continued hope.

On the very first day Dr Hilu made an agreement with Joe allowing him to continue drinking Rioja red wine (as this has fewer additives than some other wines) and whisky (as most of the sugar is turned to alcohol). In return Joe would obey the rest of the restrictions and follow the treatment. It may seem surprising that someone with cancer would need any persuasion to stick to a potentially life–saving treatment, but when cancer is diagnosed it does not come with a gift of willpower — we are all human!

On examination of Joe's blood Dr Hilu could see that his immune system was impaired. There was extensive **free radical** damage which was evidenced by white spaces within the cell structure in the blood when viewed under a microscope. His blood was also showing poor oxygenation. Oxygen in the bloodstream is extremely important as every organ in the body requires oxygen and the red blood cells provide the vehicle by which the oxygen is transported. His blood cells were all clumped together which meant that his tissues and organs were not receiving enough oxygen and his blood would not be able to carry the essential nutrients around the body and fuel it as it should. His blood was also showing signs of acidity. This is not good as the body requires a PH balance in order to maintain health and fight off diseases. (The body's ideal PH is between 7.3 and 7.45 which is slightly alkaline — values range from 1 to 14 with 1 being extremely acidic, 7 being neutral and 14 being very alkaline).

There was also evidence of metal toxicity (an excessive build–up of metals) in the body which is detrimental to health as the body has to attempt to get rid of the metals. This appeared as a dark rim on the edge of the cells within the blood. This is known to be exacerbated by the presence of amalgam fillings in the teeth. Consequently, the removal of all of Joe's amalgam fillings and replacement with white fillings was one of the first steps which we took in an effort to improve Joe's health and immune system. This was carried out by a holistic dentist (they believe in treating the whole person, will not use amalgam and believe that root canals can spread disease in the body). The removal of these fillings and the correction of any tooth problems is a vital precautionary measure as there is much evidence to show that tooth problems put an enormous constant strain on the immune system, and if the immune system is constantly fighting tooth problems how can it concentrate on fighting bigger issues i.e. cancer?

Initially we went to see Doctor Hilu every three to four months. Any changes within the blood take this long to become evident so visiting more frequently would have served no purpose. This was quite frustrating at times as we were eager to see results from the treatments which we had been following, but nature wouldn't allow our curiosity to be satisfied any sooner. However, a positive aspect was that the wait and anticipated visit gave us something on which to focus. We knew that if we did not eat healthily, if we drank too much alcohol, if we did not exercise, if we did not take our supplements, that it would be apparent in the next blood analysis and we would be in trouble.

I remember the first time that I had my blood analysed by Dr Hilu. I found it amazing that this was my blood, straight from my body, which I could see. The blood cells were various shapes and sizes, some big, some small, some strange shapes. Dr Hilu said that about fifty percent of my blood could not be doing its job correctly and that I had poor digestion, along with a lack of either vitamin B12 or folic acid. I had very bad adrenaline stress and free radical damage to my cells. I had signs of bacteria and fungus and acidic–looking blood. I was amazed as I exercised every day, ate healthily (or so I thought!) and drank moderately. I was always very busy but never really felt stressed, though I never relaxed much.

With each visit to Dr Hilu we could see the changes in our blood. In the beginning we were both very diligent and abided by all of the rules, took all of the supplements and the improvements which we could see were astonishing. However, there were times when Joe would be a naughty boy and Dr Hilu would know.

We once visited Dr Hilu in Barcelona where he has a clinic in addition to his fabulous clinic in Puerto Banus, Malaga, Spain. We were astounded to find Dr Hilu diagnosing young children who were feeling unwell with cellular medicine analysis. Their parents were using his diagnosis instead of a GP. He offers treatment with **biological therapy**. He offers various treatments including full body hyperthermia, local deep hyperthermia by radiofrequency, plasma generators, ozone therapy, colon hydrotherapy, ion transfer units, rife frequency devices, detox units, cellular analysis, and orthomolecular nutrition. He also offers tailor–made diets and his success rates make impressive reading, not only for cancer patients but for patients with other serious illnesses. I could attempt to explain all of the above but would surely fail. If you want to learn more please visit Dr Hilu's website at:

www.magnamarbellaclinic.com
email: info@magnamarbellaclinic.com.
C/Calderón de la Barca s/n, Edificio Magna Marbella, bloque Romero de Torres, 1º, 29660 Marbella (Málaga)-España. Tel.: +34 952929722. Fax: +34 952906456. Skype magnamarbellaclinic

Supplements

The supplements which Doctor Hilu recommended were as follows:–

Poly-MVA Canada

www.polymvacanada.com

Joe used to drink Poly-MVA by the bottle, sometimes consuming a quarter of a bottle in one go! He was so funny — he would pull faces because he didn't like the taste but he didn't mind — must have been because his body needed it.

Poly-MVA is a new, non-toxic, powerful **antioxidant** dietary supplement. While definitive studies on its effect in human nutrition and health are under way, early studies indicate that the active ingredients in Poly-MVA may be beneficial in protecting cell DNA , assisting the body in producing energy and providing support to the liver in removing harmful substances from the body.

Some studies indicate that ingredients of Poly-MVA can assist in preventing cell damage and removing heavy metals from the bloodstream. As a powerful antioxidant, it can help to neutralise the free radicals within the body that are thought to influence the ageing process and convert them into energy.

Poly-MVA can provide the following nutritional support to the body:

- Helps the body to produce energy
- Supports the liver in removing harmful substances from the body
- Assists in preventing cell damage
- Assists the body in removing heavy metals from the bloodstream
- Powerful antioxidant and detoxificant
- Prevents B-12 deficiency related mental disturbances in the elderly
- Supports nerve and neurotransmitter function
- Enhances white blood cell function
- Supports pH balance, helping to maintain oxygenation of cells and tissues

See Appendix 3 for full description.

Included with kind permission from Poly-MVA

Graviola

Initially we purchased graviola from Dr Hilu, but it is freely available on the internet from other sources. It is a very inexpensive supplement with astounding results. When we used it initially, Joe's PSA went down to nearly 0. We eventually stopped it as Joe's PSA was very low and very stable. We restarted it when Joe's PSA began to creep up again, and again had tremendous results with it. Graviola is a small tree with fruits of 15-20cm in length. It is cultivated in almost all of tropical America. Research has demonstrated that the acetogenins (which have similar properties to that of products used in chemotherapy such as doxorubicin with the advantage of not giving their side effects) which are found in the leaves can selectively inhibit the growth of cancer cells. There is evidence of significant achievements in the treatment of certain cancers with this plant.

Formula DEG

This supplement is manufactured by RayRos.com. It is mainly used as a natural chemotherapy backup. At the same time it reduces side–effects of cytotoxics (chemotherapy drugs) thanks to its composition: calendula, oregano, ginger, silica and magnesium. Calendula is the main active ingredient due to its anti–cancerous properties according to many experts.

For further information you can review the publications listed in Appendix 2.

COQ10

Coenzyme Q10 is an antioxidant and is found in just about every cell of the body. Electrons are transported around the body so that it can function efficiently i.e. the electrons provide energy to the body, and COQ10 is an important part of this transport system. One of the main functions of COQ10 is to help to convert food into energy. The body produces COQ10 naturally but the low levels often found in cancer patients are obviously a problem as their bodies require large amounts of antioxidants, so supplementing is a good idea.

It is reported to have many health benefits including improvement of the immune system, easing fatigue, energising the body, increasing stamina and it may improve heart health. Good sources of COQ10 are fish, beef, pork, chicken heart, chicken liver, kidney, whole grains, oily fish, peanuts and avocado. Broccoli, grapes and cauliflower also provide a smaller amount of COQ10.

Cellfood

www.nuscience.com

Cellfood is a free radical scavenger (powerful antioxidant). It helps detoxify the body and balance PH. It is made from the finest of natural, plant–based organic substances. It can be bought directly from natural product retailers and through Dr Hilu. We used Cellfood for a long period of time and I continue to use it for general health.
See Appendix 4 for full description
Included with kind permission from Nuscience

Fish Oil

Fish oil has been shown to significantly help a number of health issues. It has been shown to help prevent heart disease, reduce pain and inflammation, help to treat neurological disease, help in treating cancer, help to reverse the ageing process and improve physical and mental performance. Fish oil has been shown to reduce existing depression and improve overall mood.

Fish oil supplements, such as salmon oil, contain omega–3 fatty acids, essential fats that decrease harmful inflammation in the body's tissues and reduce the risk of chronic diseases. Fish oil is a rich source of omega–3 fatty acids EPA (eicosapentaenoic acid) and DHA (docosahexaenoic acid). It has been discovered that EPA interferes with the inflammatory mechanisms that cause loss of muscle mass. In addition, a number of experimental studies have shown that fish oil, particularly DHA, can boost the responsiveness to chemotherapy and radiotherapy and that a diet rich in fish oil tends to slow tumour growth, partly due to its suppressive effect on angiogenesis (the process by which new blood vessels develop to enable the growth and spread of tumours). Fish oil also has the ability to help fend off cachexia (the severe loss of muscle mass that often complicates late stage cancer).

One must, however, be very careful to choose the best quality product. Fish oil is inexpensive and readily available on the internet and in natural product retailer stores.

Formula Immune

Formula Immune contains arabinogalactans (which are basically large molecules produced by living organisms) and non–acidifying vitamin C. Arabinogalactans have been highly researched both as prebiotics and immune system boosters as well as anti–cancer supplements.

See Appendix 5 for full description

Oxygen Treatment

During a visit to Dr Hilu he checked Joe's oxygen level in his blood and found it to be a little low. He measured this with a pulse oximeter which is a small device that fits onto the finger and measures the pulse and also the oxygen levels in the blood. This is quite a useful device and we always owned one of these — they are readily available on the internet. Low oxygen in the blood can be common in cancer patients as the lactic acid build–up around the cancer cells prevents the transport of oxygen into neighbouring cells. Cancer cells don't like oxygen. They are partially anaerobic (they rely more on the glucose in cells for their energy than oxygen).

Dr Hilu had a portable oxygen machine in his clinic which he kindly allowed us to purchase. The model was a Bol d'Air from Holiste Laboratoires in France. Joe used it every day. I do believe that he benefited from it, particularly towards the end when he got quite breathless, especially after chemotherapy treatments.

We discovered another place for oxygen therapy at the West Yorkshire Multiple Sclerosis Therapy Centre. Apparently, clinical trials have been carried out indicating that for multiple sclerosis sufferers there was an improvement in symptoms and protection from deterioration by breathing pure oxygen whilst under increased air pressure.

The centre has different tanks similar to diving tanks and you can choose to experience going to different depths depending on the condition of your health. Joe went there at least once a week in the last two or three years of his illness. I would say that he always felt much better after having been there.

There remains much controversy surrounding the benefits of oxygen therapy. Some supporters claim that cancer cells thrive in low oxygen environments and they believe that by adding oxygen to the body, an oxygen rich condition is created in which cancer cells cannot survive. It is claimed that it increases the efficiency of all of the cells in the body, thereby increasing energy and promoting the production of antioxidants.

Oxygen therapy has many other uses including reducing tissue damage and side–effects when used with radiotherapy and improving the uptake of chemotherapy drugs.

The Role of Hyperthermia in the battle against Cancer

There are more than fifty–five thousand scientific publications that should encourage oncologists to utilise this powerful tool which involves elevating the tumour's temperature up till 42'9 ºC for one hour for ten days. Cancer cells are thermo–sensitive and thus easily destroyed by high temperature.

See Appendix 2 for bibliography

Included with kind permission from Dr Hilu

The Papimi Machine

www.papimi.com

Unfortunately this is definitely not affordable for the majority of people as it costs around £35,000, but we felt that it was well worth the investment as it should preferably be used for a period of time so we bought our own machine and imported it from Greece.

The Papimi — NanoPulse Therapy system is a medical device producing electromagnetic pulses, invented by the Greek Professor Dr Panos Pappas. It restores the electric potential of the cells, which in turn regulates the chemical interchanges towards normality in instances of disequilibrium. In other words it brings the body's electro–magnetic field back into balance.

See Appendix 6 for full description

Included with kind permission from Papimi.com

Budwig Diet

We were advised by Dr Hilu to research the Budwig diet. It wasn't something that he insisted that we follow, but we did analyse whether we felt that it would be a good diet for us at the time. Because we were so focused on the cellular medicine analysis and the supplements which Dr Hilu had given to us we decided that it may interfere with our aims at that time. Also, this treatment does not sit well with vitamin C infusions which Joe was having.

Dr Johanna Budwig was seven times nominated for the Nobel Prize in Medicine. During her investigations she discovered the powerful healing nature of essential fatty acids in many degenerative diseases, including cancer. She wrote numerous books that reflect the critical importance of polyunsaturated fatty acids and the negative effect of toxic trans–hydrogenated fats (processed by having hydrogen pumped through them at high temperatures and used in margarines, cooking oils etc.) and saturated fats on health. Her studies produced research that indicates that the imbalance of electro–chemicals transforms healthy cells into cancer cells.

The diet is based on flaxseed oil, cottage cheese and naturally occurring foods. Although I say that we didn't follow it, the list of recommended foods is almost exactly the list of foods which we allowed in our diet.

It would also seem that the scientific world has taken the findings regarding the use of flaxseed oil in the treatment of certain cancers on board and scientists have had some very positive results in initial research tests. However, the results from these trials are a long way from being published and accepted as fact.

For full details of the diet see the website:

www.budwigcenter.com/

Included with kind permission from the Budwig Center

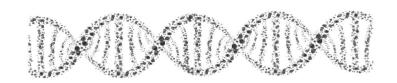

6 — Professor Oliver

Meeting Professor Oliver — Also known as Prof

I read everything that I could about prostate cancer: alternative cures, conventional cures, specialists and professors of oncology. I came across some very nice and helpful specialists and professors and was amazed at how they took the time to talk to me and help me. I became aware of a very helpful gentleman who spoke to me by telephone from his hospital bed whilst recovering from an operation. I later found out that this man was one of the members of the scientific advisory board for Life Extension (_www.lef.org_) and co-founder and past medical director of the Prostate Cancer Research Institute. He very kindly recommended Professor Oliver at St Barts Hospital, London. The gentleman advised that he had heard that Professor Oliver was extremely knowledgeable in his field and that he was doing some very good work in treating prostate cancer with intermittent hormone therapy. We located Professor Oliver and arranged to meet him on the 21st November 2005.

Professor Oliver is a wonderful man. He helped Joe and I with all of our medical needs and questions. He was always interested to know about our alternative cures and encouraged us to explore alternative options, although he emphasised the importance of robust data before beginning. It is difficult to find a doctor — in this case a professor of oncology — who agrees with trying alternative treatments. Sometimes, however, he would ask that we adhere only to his medication for a while so that he could accurately assess which treatments were working. He advised that trying too many treatments together could mask which one was actually being effective or even worse nullify the effect of one that does work. He was, of course, correct. I was eager to try everything but sometimes this did make it difficult to see exactly which treatment was having the positive/negative effect.

Professor Oliver is co-founder of the Orchid Cancer Research charity (www.orchid-cancer.org.uk). It is a UK registered cancer charity which focuses entirely on the male–specific cancers: prostate, penile and testicular. They offer support and information to people affected by, or interested in, male cancer through a dedicated medical research programme, education and awareness campaigns and a range of support services. Professor Oliver has now retired from Orchid.

Professor Oliver focused on hormone treatments including anti–androgen treatments. Hormones are produced naturally in the body and act as chemical messengers, passing instructions to cells and organs. Without testosterone, a male sex hormone, most prostate cancers cannot grow. Anti–androgen and hormone therapies work to interfere with the production of male sex hormones, or to change the instructions which they are passing on. Professor Oliver's view was that once the PSA has come down sufficiently from the effects of the treatment the patient should have a break and wait until the PSA starts to rise again before restarting. In this way, the hormone therapy is likely to continue to be effective over a longer period of time, and by providing drug–free time the patient has chance to feel 'normal' again and regain some of their sex drive. Joe's case was a little different from the usual case as his PSA was always low, at least for the first five years, even though the cancer was a very aggressive type. The PSA never went above 10 in the first five years which is extremely unusual with aggressive metastatic disease.

We initially started with blood tests to monitor the cancer every three months. We then changed it to every month, then every two weeks and sometimes every week when the PSA was increasing or a new treatment was being introduced. When the PSA was doubling in a matter of weeks, even days, we knew that this potentially spelt trouble. Unfortunately for National Health patients, regular blood tests are not always so easily available. As Joe was a private patient I could request blood tests as often as was deemed necessary when the cancer was not stable, or after an onset of pain as this would usually indicate another **flare**.

Joe continued to be administered three–monthly goserelin injections until we met Professor Oliver who stopped them. Joe was really happy about this as he had consistently said that he thought that they weren't necessary and that they caused him to be depressed and tearful. They had also caused him to gain weight. When Professor

Oliver said that he could stop taking it Joe boasted that he had been correct about not needing the injections. Who can say — they can't have done any harm and in the early stages of treatment it is better to try too much than too little.

The amazing result was that from this point Joe managed to remain free from any treatment, apart from alternative ones, for three years. This was truly remarkable with such advanced metastatic disease. He managed to live for seven years after his cancer was found. Who knows for how long he had been suffering? Had he been a more obedient patient then I am sure that he could have carried on for longer.

In April 2008, following a visit to a clinic in Mexico, the cancer became more active. Professor Oliver (Prof) advised Joe to restart hormone therapy treatment consisting of a different drug called **flutamide**, an oral, non-steroidal drug. Flutamide is one of the oldest anti-androgens and is said to have more side-effects, but Joe was quite tolerant of this one. Later, in July 2008, his PSA rose again. Joe was once again prescribed bicalutamide which he had previously been taking before the prostatectomy. At the end of September, the PSA again rose and the decision was taken to revert to goserelin which had been prescribed in the beginning by Professor Jones. Second time round goserelin was effective for about nine months. Joe was given monthly injections so that his progress could be more closely monitored. In December 2008 **zoledronic acid** infusions were added to strengthen his bones. This was administered in our home by 'Healthcare at Home' nurses (www.hah.co.uk). They are a private healthcare group who can carry out certain medical procedures — blood tests, infusions etc. in the home. I always found the nurses to be very compassionate and professional. We paid for this service and the zoledronic acid purely because it provided comfort for Joe to be cared for at home. However, the same treatment was available free at the hospital. Little did we know that there are extremely dangerous possible complications with **bisphosphonates**, of which zoledronic acid is one, such as osteonecrosis of the jaw.

In April 2009 Joe was admitted briefly for pain control and Joe's pain and PSA responded very rapidly to **diethylstilbestrol** and **dexamethasone**. Unfortunately, the response was short-lived and in June 2009, six weeks later, he had a further pain recurrence after a long air flight and was admitted as an emergency to a hospital in London. Joe was in agony, close to screaming he was in so much pain. We were scared as we did not know what was causing such agony and we feared the worst. Finally, Prof administered steroids and the pain settled. We slept together in a single camp bed on the floor in the hospital, squeezing each other so hard as if never to let go, wondering what tomorrow would bring. The pain did not completely go away and we knew that we had to do something quickly, but what?

Prof suggested an oral chemotherapy which was available on a trial study. He told us that we could still travel and live a normal life with this so it was the best option. We agreed — we trusted Prof implicitly and knew that he would not recommend chemotherapy unless it was the only option left. It was still a shock as we knew that our options were now running out. We had never wanted chemotherapy to be part of Joe's treatment, but at this stage there was nowhere else to go. I feared that once we started down the chemotherapy path that it was the path to the end of Joe's life, and I was right.

Firstly Joe was prescribed **chlorambucil** and **lomustine** but unfortunately this did not work well and he was soon suffering a lot of pain. The PSA had now escalated to over 100. Prof started Joe on **docetaxel** chemotherapy. This kept the cancer under control only for about six weeks, and then he added **carboplatin** (intra–venous) and the results were very positive. The PSA came all the way down to 4. Joe's condition improved and the cancer settled for a while. Prof added **degarelix** and yet again we achieved results. It was like a game of chess, constantly attempting to out–manoeuvre the enemy, with the joys of success and the despair of the failures.

In January 2010 Joe suddenly developed double vision.

'I can see two of you darling!' he laughed. Nothing phased Joe, even though he could not drive anywhere or go anywhere unaided. We went to London for a scan which revealed a cavernous sinus thrombosis (a blood clot which forms in the cavernous sinus which sits at the base of the brain and is life–threatening) which had developed from a skull base metastases (the cancer spreading to the base of the skull). Professor Oliver was very attentive, always quick to try something else when the cancer started to pick up pace. He started Joe back on diethylstilbestrol and dexamethasone, which gave some relief to the problem, and he was immediately on the case with a suggestion of **gamma knife treatment**. To have the gamma knife treatment Joe had to have a steel cage screwed into his skull. I almost fainted when I saw him! He said it didn't hurt — gosh, what a brave man he was. The cage was to ensure that the radiation beam would hit exactly the right spot and there would be no movement or mistakes. Thankfully all went smoothly and soon Joe's vision was back to normal. When he came back from the procedure, as a reward for his bravery, I had been to Harrods and bought him the biggest crab ever and we had our little seafood party in the hospital to celebrate. Small wins become big celebrations in this fight.

After this episode of double vision we travelled to the Maldives for a break. We were still trying to keep our lives as normal as possible and travel was a large part of our normal activity. Whilst we were there Joe developed vertigo and could not come out of the room for most of the time. Constant dizziness prevented him from even getting up from the bed. Again I gave him some steroids and the doctor gave him some tablets for vertigo, but these did not help much. During our stay in the Maldives Joe's health had deteriorated fast. We felt that all options in the UK had been exhausted. Following much research we decided to head to the Cancer Clinic in Houston.

Included with kind permission from Professor Oliver

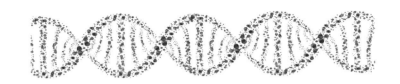

7 — Dr Hilbert Seeger

Meeting Dr Seeger

It was October 2008 and we had spent a long summer on the boat in the sunshine. I spent most of the time by Joe's side and I can tell you that I am so happy now that I did. Our times together were so precious.

We ate healthily on the boat, buying fresh, locally caught fish, organic fruit and locally produced vegetables where possible.

I remained keen to learn more about the blood and its analysis, and I stumbled across an advert on the internet for a forthcoming medical exhibition in Germany. Attending would be a few live blood doctors, some of them medical experts, famous worldwide, so I decided to go. Joe decided to come with me, which was unexpected as it wasn't his sort of thing, but I was pleased that he did.

We stayed in the picturesque, quaint town of Baden Baden. At the exhibition there were several demonstrations on live blood analysis. I had previously contacted an amiable doctor called Dr Hilbert Seeger. He was something of an expert on live blood analysis and we arranged to meet him at the show.

We quickly found Dr Seeger and introduced ourselves. We chatted about my research and, as he was set up ready to perform live blood analysis, he offered to do our bloods as a demonstration. My blood was all clumped together which, he explained, was probably due to the flying and dehydration. He was selling DVDs on how to practice live blood analysis and offering a question and answer helpline to help practitioners learn how to perform it. This would have been an excellent support network had I taken my interest further and started to practice, but keeping Joe alive was the main priority and everything else had to wait.

I asked if he could teach me more on live blood analysis. Joe, who was normally one step ahead of me, said 'Why don't you come to visit us Dr Seeger? You can teach Julie and stay with us'. Much to my surprise, Hilbert agreed immediately and gave me his available dates, which were as soon as the following week.

Vitamin C

Dr Seeger arrived, as promised, in England. I invited friends, family and employees to my home to have live blood analysis performed by him. He also did his own blood, which was perfect! During his visit I increased my knowledge extensively.

Whilst Hilbert was with us, he gave Joe a high dose of intravenous vitamin C every other day. The actual process was highly amusing — Hilbert had the drip assembled on a coat hanger hooked over a light fitting high up on the wall. He wanted to teach me how to administer the vitamin C intravenously, but I was too afraid to do it. We were advised at the beginning to avoid vitamin C infusions whilst having chemotherapy as it may lessen the effects of the chemotherapy. However, more recent studies have indicated that it may be more beneficial than detrimental to have it alongside chemotherapy. Also, research indicates that, at high doses and used in conjunction with chemotherapy or radiation, it helps to kill early stage cancer and strengthens the immune system.

Unfortunately, it is very difficult to find anywhere in England to administer high doses of vitamin C intravenously although it is easy to find in many other countries. I eventually found a place in Greater Manchester which we visited every fortnight. It was a clinic mainly for heart patients who went to receive **chelation therapy** to clean their arteries and veins. Joe would have high dose vitamin C, DMSO and niacin.

Joe loved his trips to Manchester. The infusion gave him renewed energy and a feeling of well-being immediately following it and he very much believed in it. The treatment generally took about an hour once Joe was 'hooked up' as Mark, the director of the clinic, would say. The clinic was a large, detached mansion house, huddled on a main road with a small car park at the end of a short driveway. Inside the atmosphere was relaxed and homely, with two sitting rooms furnished with mis-matched but comfortable chairs and drip stands which were scattered around. Most of Mark's patients were over sixty and some had been visiting him for over ten years. Mark's wife would run around with cups of tea and biscuits for everyone. The only downside to the treatment was the terrible garlic smell from the DMSO which Joe was left with afterwards. I can remember being in the car on the journey home from the clinic — the smell was terrible. It usually lingered for at least the next day also, although in all honesty it did not bother me as long as it was doing some good.

We would always call for our Costa coffee on the way home — maybe subconsciously to try to get rid of the smell! I encouraged Joe to drink a daily coffee as more and more research is indicating that coffee has many benefits, one of which is that it makes chemotherapy more effective, and it has antioxidant properties. The key is not to overindulge. Everything in moderation.

Doctor Seeger's Input

I felt that it was very important that the work of Doctor Seeger should not be misrepresented in any way. Therefore, Doctor Seeger kindly contributed a document which can be found at Appendix 1 as it may be rather technical for some readers, but I feel that it adds value for those interested in the scientific explanations of the causes of cancer.

Summary of this Period

My knowledge was greatly improved by spending time with Dr Seeger and Dr Hilu and by taking the courses which I attended in Chicago for live blood analysis. I also attended a course on flow analysis (the analysis of the body fluids including saliva, urine, water and blood), which, when used in conjunction with the live blood analysis, enables one to make a very accurate diagnosis of the imbalances and problems within a patient.

I took Joe's blood constantly throughout his illness and could see when I needed to make changes to his alternative medicine. I never stuck to the same alternative treatment for any period of time but continually changed it and added different treatments. Cancer is very clever and can become resistant to many things with which you attack it, so it is better to keep trying different treatments in order to surprise the enemy.

Towards the end, the free radical damage to the cells was unbelievably extensive. The whole cell was almost totally white instead of red, white on the cell being the evidence of free radical damage.

I discussed with Dr Seeger the possibility of going to another clinic, perhaps another one in Mexico where we had already been. Dr Seeger said that he would not recommend Mexico as, in his opinion, many of the clinics are a rip–off and don't help, but he did recommend that we should try the Paracelsus Clinic in Switzerland. He told us that he personally knew one of the doctors there and, in his opinion, it was a good clinic and better than the clinics in Mexico. So, on his recommendation, we decided to go.

Included with kind permission from Dr Seeger

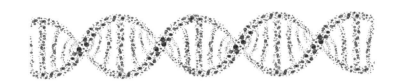

8 — Visits to Clinics

Why We Visited Alternative Therapy Clinics

The clinics which we visited have mixed reviews from the medical world and the media, but when Joe was diagnosed the cancer within his body and bones was at an advanced stage so it was an easy decision for us to try everything which afforded a chance, however small, of extending his life with some measure of quality and health. However, each person must assess every piece of information about the treatments available and how effective they may be on their particular cancer. Most of the treatments are not supported by approved clinical trials, so the individual does not have the comfort of knowing that someone 'in the know' has passed the treatments as 'safe'. However, after weighing up all of the information available to me, we decided to visit the following clinics. In most instances I wish that I had known about these clinics earlier. It may then be that I could have kept my wonderful husband alive for longer. As it was, I firmly believe that the treatments which he received extended his life for months and years. The clinics, costing thousands of pounds apart from the Essaidi Aqua Tilis Therapy, are beyond many people's budgets, but how much does one day, one week, one year of life cost? For me, every penny was well spent. I believe that we learnt much from our visits to the clinics, even if sometimes the learning was about our strengths and weaknesses rather than about the extension of life.

I hope that you will find our travels informative and that our experiences and the information here may help people to make the right decisions regarding alternative cancer treatments for themselves or their loved ones, but **only** after consultation with your medical practitioner.

The Essaidi Aqua Tilis Therapy

www.essaidi.nl

A friend of a friend told us about a clinic in Eindhoven, not far from Amsterdam, which was curing people of various diseases. I quickly investigated and we decided to give it a try.

We first visited the clinic in April 2005. The founder's daughter runs the clinic, a clean and modest structure which exudes an air of quiet confidence and friendliness. The founder and inventor of the clinic and therapy makes a point of welcoming new visitors and is proficient at remembering names — this was also the doctor with whom we initially had an appointment. After we had explained about Joe's cancer, he advised that he would make up a special detox medicine for Joe which would compliment his cancer treatment.

The therapy is designed to eradicate free radical damage to cells and to stimulate the production of new cells. The treatment helps to repair DNA, strengthen the immune system, improve oxygenation and reduce inflammation. Hundreds of patients have been treated with the Essaidi Method and had tremendous results.

You could describe the treatment as an incredibly hot steam room. It was unexpected how it sapped the body of energy, especially on our first visit there. After the treatment you feel absolutely wonderful, revitalised, refreshed and renewed. It is possible for two people to share a cabin together if the patient needs assistance or is at all apprehensive — I shared a cabin with Joe to begin with, but we soon realised that in Joe's case this was not necessary.

We hired bikes whilst we were in Eindhoven and cycled from our hotel to the clinic and back every day, a round journey of about an hour. On our first trip to the clinic, we did one session per day. However, on subsequent trips Joe decided that we could do two sessions in the day, which was absolutely fine in the beginning, but towards the end this proved a little challenging for him. We visited the clinic twice during the year and did so for a few years but we only visited once in the final year due to Joe's health.

I would truly recommend this treatment. I still go myself once a year and I really look forward to the visit. It works as a good detox and immune system strengthener for me.

The best description of the treatment is given below by kind courtesy of Hanna, the daughter of the creator of the therapy:

Mr. Essaidi was working at Phillips medical system as a

developer of medical devices. During his study in Moscow he learned a lot about physics and the human body. In 1988 he built the first cabin with his knowledge. The cabin is a pyramid shaped room and the room is covered in mirrors. The mirror's function is to reflect the lights in the room. Behind the mirrors are coils and speakers to create a magnetic field and fibration. The frequency of the magnetic field is programmed on the illness that someone has. There is steam in the room and the temperature varies from low to high. This is to promote the blood circulation and to detox the body. In the cabin there is also a package of oxygen to relax the breathing.

The Aqua Tilis Therapy uses physics based terms to influence undesirable reactions and information–relay within the human body. The therapy analyses processes within the human body, not only from a biological and chemical perspective, as is the case in conventional medical science, but also from a physics perspective. Using this approach we can apply know–how from the classic electro– and atom physics to, for example, change characteristics of metabolic processes or influence frequencies of nerve impulses. Even though these principles are well known in the field of physics they are seldom applied in bio–medical science.

When referring to 'normal' biochemical reactions and signals, we should realise that these are defined under the 'normal' conditions of the electromagnetic field surrounding the Earth. When the electromagnetic field around a living organism is altered, that will have consequences for the structure and the behaviour of molecules and cells in that organism. Space travel provides a good example of this: the altered electromagnetic field surrounding the astronauts (the loss of gravity which causes weightlessness) causes, amongst others things, the metabolic pattern in the bones to change so much that it ultimately results in osteoporosis. This is one of the leading medical challenges that long–term space travel is faced with. Furthermore, it is also generally known that the dissolvability of substances (e.g. calcium deposits) can be changed by modulating electromagnetic fields.

With regard to certain medical problems e.g. broken bones, the positive effects of using electromagnetic fields to assist healing has been recognised for years; with regard to orthopaedic and pain related treatments the TENS–principle (transepidermal neurostimulation) has been applied for many years.

The Aqua Tilis Therapy makes selective use of specific

electromagnetic fields to modulate certain bodily functions. These electromagnetic fields can be specifically defined (frequency, strength, etc.) and the physiological effects measured objectively.

The Aqua Tilis Therapy focuses on situations where a process within the human body has gone wrong forming the basis for chronic illness. An important role in this procedure is known as 'oxidative stress'. Oxidative stress can be caused by external factors e.g. air pollution, infection, incorrect nutrition, obesity, smoking, etc. However, it is not always possible to ascertain whether oxidative stress is the cause or the result of a process in the body which has gone wrong. Either way, combating oxidative stress has a positive effect and usually leads to an improvement of the state of health of the patient.

Oxidative stress leads to an excessive exchange of electrons between molecules in cells and tissue. The elements involved in this process are called 'free radicals'. They draw away electrons from substances which they come in contact with. Under normal circumstances free radicals help to regulate blood pressure and stimulate activity of the immune system. They are kept under control by anti–radicals or antioxidants which are present in proper (healthy) food and as a result of a healthy life–style with plenty of exercise (cells will then be able to 'arm' themselves sufficiently against free radicals in the body). Oxidative stress causes a slowdown of the body's counteraction of free radicals resulting in an excessive exchange of electrons (oxidation process). This 'electron storm' can cause damage to cell membranes, to DNA, etc. This in turn results in certain genes being activated and others deactivated. Ultimately this can result in a chronic stimulation of the body's defence system, the immune system, with its links to the nerve and hormone systems. 'Chronic Immune Stimulation' is the basis for many chronic diseases such as heart and artery diseases, neuro–degenerative diseases, cancer, lung disease and auto–immune diseases e.g. rheumatism.

One of the goals of the Aqua Tilis Therapy is to counteract and ultimately stop oxidative stress and the related pathological reactions. This is realised by using different related technologies.

The sauna style cabin is kept at a relatively high humidity and a temperature of around 50°C. The effects of the high humidity and temperature of a sauna on the human body are well known and not disputed; during transpiration (transfer of water to the atmosphere), the skin is used as a supportive organ to the neutralisation and disposal of unwanted chemicals including free radicals. The atmosphere in the cabin contains an excessive (and objectively measurable) positive charge, which is achieved by a special type of electrolysis of water contained in a reservoir in the cabin. Moving electromagnets behind the mirrored walls of the cabin create the specific magnetic fields required to allow the positively charged particles in the cabin's atmosphere to neutralise the excess of negative charge which is caused by oxidative stress. The moving electromagnets can be combined with static magnets which can be placed within the cabin. These combined fields also assist the dissolvability of deposits (e.g. calcium deposits in arteries) and improve circulation in general.

Certain frequencies can also have an anti-microbial effect. By using so-called resonance-frequencies, bacteria, moulds and viruses can be counteracted. This resonance-frequency mechanism can be demonstrated by a platoon of soldiers marching across a bridge. They must fall out of step in case the resonance frequency of their marching matches that of the bridge and destroys it.

Another aspect of the Aqua Tilis Therapy technology focuses on modulating signals between the brain and the body's organs. Each brain signal has a specific frequency. This also applies to pain signals. Knowledge of these specific frequencies opens up the possibilities of counteracting or altogether stopping pain or other signals.

All the functions of the Aqua Tilis Therapy cabin are fully integrated and are monitored by a computer system. This means that, at any time during the treatment, they can be adjusted to meet specific individual needs.

Aqua Tilis Therapy:

- Neutralises and removes chemicals and organisms (free radicals, microbes, etc.) related to illness and disease from the body
- Intensifies immune cell activity and increases the efficiency of the blood circulation
- Gives the normal physiology of the human body a chance to recover
- Stimulates blood circulation
- Detoxifies organs (detox)
- Helps the nervous system and with oxidative stress

- Corrects signalling of the brain to spinal cord
- Stabilizes free radicals
- Provides supportive therapy in cancer, neurological disorders and urological disorders
- Improves skin condition
- Facilitates and strengthens joints
- Improves body condition
- Reduces old medication

Included with kind permission from Hanna, Essaidi Aqua Tilis Therapy

On one occasion, after leaving the clinic we went straight to Spain and had our blood analysed under a microscope by Dr Hilu. He asked what we had been doing as all of our free radicals were on the outside of the cells. We explained that we had just been to the Essaidi Aqua Tilis Therapy and he nodded his understanding of what he was seeing. The free radicals were being pushed out of the cells and the cells were repairing and renewing. He advised that we should continue to use the sauna for another couple of weeks to help to complete the treatment.

Joe always had his own sauna which he enjoyed immensely and he would take a sauna every other day when we were home. A sauna helps the detoxifying process and helps to remove toxins from the body through sweat — indeed, saunas can have many health benefits. An infrared sauna is different to a normal sauna in that it uses infrared heaters to emit infrared radiant heat which is absorbed by the surface of the skin; traditional saunas heat the body primarily by conduction and convection from the heated air and by radiation of the heated surfaces in the sauna room. Therefore, when entering the infrared sauna it does not feel hot. It is a completely different experience to the normal sauna where you can sometimes feel the heat is too much when inside. However, you sweat exactly the same and the benefits of the infrared sauna are said to be as good if not better. Joe preferred the normal sauna to the infrared sauna. He loved the heat and could stand a really high temperature, but he did use both and would always sleep a lot better afterwards.

Alternative Medicine Clinic Mexico

We were strong advocates of cellular medicine analysis, believing that it provided a valuable insight as to whether treatments were working or not as changes in the cells were visible evidence of progress, and I was very keen to learn more on the subject. I found an American company which offered courses in blood microscopy and flow analysis. Having booked onto the blood microscopy course, I learned of a gentleman who was practicing this close to us in the UK. We decided to pay him a visit to find out whether he was offering the same service as Dr Hilu in Spain. He was performing blood microscopy, together with a general checkup — checking the heart, the urine and the saliva — a very similar service to the flow analysis which I learnt in Chicago.

During our visit to the gentleman in the UK, he told us of a clinic in Mexico and strongly recommended that we should visit. He said that he had recommended it to many clients and that great results were being achieved, especially with cancer patients. He believed that Joe's health could be deteriorating according to his cellular medicine analysis results and the slightly rising PSA.

I would try anything and everything to keep Joe alive for longer and so we immediately made plans to go. I had a courageous patient who, with my encouragement, was extremely willing to co-operate, which made all of my efforts worthwhile. I had seen no signs to indicate that Joe's condition was worsening at this stage although his PSA was rising very slightly and, considering his diagnosis, I knew that the cancer would never go away, so I was always looking for the next plan, the next alternative treatment, the next way of outsmarting the cancer. I lived and breathed it. Every day there would be a new problem.

Fortunately it was not so busy at the clinic and they had room for us in two weeks time so in the third week of March 2008 we travelled to Mexico, flying to San Diego, California. We were met by a driver who escorted us to the Mexican border, where we had to stop to get a visa. There were hundreds of people selling things at the border on the roadside and many people crossing through, even on foot.

Across the border from San Diego there are approximately fifty clinics offering alternative cancer treatments for fees that can run into tens of thousands of dollars which are not allowed to operate within the USA as the treatments have not been approved by the FDA (Food and Drugs Administration). This particular clinic was a modern–looking building. It had an outpatients department, many inpatient rooms and an adjoining pharmacy. We were shown around the building and then to our room which was no more than a hospital room with a hospital bed and one single bed for me. After settling into the room we sampled the food, which was fabulous — an Aladdin's cave of fresh, organic fruit and vegetables. There was always some protein, either fish or chicken and a rice, bean or cereal dish, but I don't recall seeing any red meat. There were no oranges — when I asked why I was told that they did not allow oranges as they were not good for cancer patients as they were too acidic.

Joe's programme was intense with infusions most days. It was towards the end of the first week before any scans were carried out on Joe as there was no availability until that time. This, in hindsight, could have been detrimental to the treatment programme and the progression of Joe's cancer as, when the scans came back, they showed that the cancer was active. I wondered if this could have been made worse due to the radiation from flying and the accompanying stress of being away from home. Perhaps it was due to the alternative treatment protocol (plan for a course of medical treatment) or a combination of everything? The fact that the PSA was rising corroborated the findings.

After the first week of treatment, we escaped for the weekend to San Diego. Not long into the trip Joe suddenly experienced extreme pain and could not even walk. He spent the following morning in bed, getting up for a few hours but then having to go back to bed in the afternoon. The second day he was a little better but still had pain.

On Monday we were back in the clinic for more treatment. The doctors came with the PSA results which had risen further and once again there was cancer activity showing on the scans. Joe continued with the same treatment for another week. He was very bored in the clinic, the highlight of each day being meal times. We were allowed out of the clinic when Joe did not have any treatments scheduled and we would go to the beach which was an eerie, wide stretch of emptiness, the promenade resembling something from the Wild West just before the outlaws hit town. We bought fresh coconuts from a stall by the beach and drank the fresh juice.

The weather was glorious so whilst Joe was having treatment I decided to go for a run. I had been assured by the clinic that it was safe to run on the beach close by. As I headed towards the beach, the streets were completely deserted, like a ghost town. There were quite a few people on one side of the beach, but one side of the beach was completely empty. I decided to run there, being careful not to run too far in case someone followed me. Within five minutes I was surrounded by jeeps!

'Put your hands above your head,' a big, chunky lady in uniform shouted. 'What are you doing?'

'I am going for a run,' I replied.

'You have just crossed the border to America. Where is your passport?'

'I don't have it. It's back at the hospital where I am staying with my sick husband.'

One policeman took pity on me, thank goodness! I had not seen any signs for the border — no wonder everyone had been looking at me strangely as I jogged by. Thankfully the policeman understood my mistake but the big woman was ready to see me behind bars. They finally let me go and told me not to cross again without my passport. What a relief! As I made my way back towards the clinic, a car pulled up alongside me and crawled along at my running pace. There were a couple of men inside who were trying to get my attention. I was very scared and took refuge beside some stands where people were selling food and drink where I waited for about ten minutes until I saw the car disappear. I then sped as fast as I could down the never-ending, deserted road back to the clinic. I don't think I've ever run so fast in my life! That was the last time that I ran alone.

Joe decided that he would learn to speak Italian whilst he was at the clinic. It was hilarious. He bought some beginners CDs. I chuckle to myself as I write this, crying and laughing as I remember him repeating the Italian phrases: benvenuto, buongiorno — bonjourno, ciao — chow, arrivederci — ahrreevaydayrchee, si — see. He did not get very far. He made me laugh so much that my sides hurt.

During our stay we conversed with some of the patients. There was a teenage girl who had a severe form of leukaemia — she had visited the clinic before and seemed happy so far with her results. There was also a young woman in her thirties — she had never smoked, was slim and health conscious and she had cancer of the lung. She had a blog on the internet which I followed for a while — later when I looked her up she was nowhere to be found.

Many of the patients were evidently very sick which showed in their appearance. Talking to one of them I was disturbed to be told that they were under the impression that, because of my appearance, I was the patient and not Joe. I hadn't realised how bad I looked due to carrying the strain of my sick husband on my shoulders; thin, frail, gaunt, worried and under constant strain, but it was a small price to pay to know that Joe never had to spend a minute thinking about his cancer treatment as I always had everything under control. You have to fight continually and never let your guard down when faced with cancer.

For many, the clinic was obviously their last hope. This was definitely not our last hope — our visit was just a continuation of our battle. In general everyone looked sick apart from one man who was bouncing around telling everyone how the clinic had cured him. He had suffered with lung cancer but was in remission and had been symptom-free for ten years or more. He lived just over the border in America. Joe thought that he was paid to visit the clinic to make everyone believe that the treatment worked and to promote business. Who knows? I believe that the clinic has helped a lot of people and cured some people. Every case is different and what works for one person does not always work in the same way for another.

Treatments at the clinic were mainly carried out using alternative medicine in conjunction with conventional medicine i.e. chemotherapy. Joe's treatment was meant to be using alternative treatment only. We didn't realise at the time, but Joe's treatment *did* include chemotherapy as it included the treatments 'cytoxic therapy and oxidative pre-conditioning and immune therapy'. To be honest, things were not explained very explicitly and we were very much in their hands. Why did I accept the treatments which we were given then and not question as doggedly as I had in the UK with the NHS doctors? I'm not sure. Perhaps it was because we were prepared to try anything that wouldn't actually kill him and we believed that any natural or alternative therapy would only improve things.

I believe that when they reviewed the severity of Joe's condition following the scans they realised that there was no option but to use the alternative treatments in conjunction with chemotherapy as they would be ineffective on their own. Whilst at the clinic Joe had been given infusions of **amygdalin** which is made from crushed apricot pits and is meant to reduce cancer's resistance to treatment and releases cyanide to kill cancer cells directly. Later when Joe was found to have high levels of cyanide in his blood, doctors looked at me with suspicion, but fortunately they knew that I was only trying to save him and had used amygdalin. In America, just over the border, amygdalin is banned as it is not FDA approved. However, this clinic believed it to be an effective treatment.

In the treatment protocol Joe also had infusions of mega doses of vitamin C together with infusions of an oxygen carrier. Vitamin C has now been proved as an effective alternative cancer treatment and helps to keep the immune system boosted.

Joe had sessions of ozone–AHT and UV light blood irradiation. This involved taking some of his blood out and treating it with a mixture of ozone and oxygen and re–infusing it. Apparently this protocol has been used in Europe for decades with an excellent safety record.

Joe received many supplements which he was to take on a daily basis, which were as follows:

Melatonin

Melatonin is a natural hormone and antioxidant produced primarily by the pineal gland at the base of the brain. As we begin to fall asleep, the body automatically gives us a burst of melatonin to aid sleep and keep our bodily rhythms in time. It has been tested in clinical trials in a wide range of cancers. Sometimes it is used as a stand–alone treatment in patients for whom further chemotherapy is not an option and sometimes it is used to help to make the chemotherapy or radiation more effective, also relieving some of the side–effects. It is best to administer melatonin at night as this is when the body would normally do so. The production of melatonin declines as the body ages and so supplements may be beneficial for older people anyway. Joe used it whilst he was in the clinic and indeed he did sleep quite well. He continued to use it from time to time when he struggled to sleep.

Silibinin

Recent studies over the last decades suggest that Silibinin can help to slow the multiplication of cancer cells by making them more susceptible to the killing effects of chemotherapy. It is also said to increase the rate of **apoptosis.**

Selenium

Selenium is an important antioxidant nutrient that supports the productions of enzymes that protect our cells against oxidant stress. This is important as oxidants can damage DNA, leading to potentially carcinogenic mutations. Although selenium alone isn't effective as a cancer therapy, supplemental selenium can render cancer cells more sensitive to chemotherapy and radiation, help to minimize chemotherapy side-effects and help to strengthen the immune system to fight the spread of cancer.

After Leaving the Clinic in Mexico

When the time came to leave the clinic, we were most certainly ready. We took enough vitamins with us to last for a couple of weeks and injections of amygdalin and chemotherapy tablets. We were not too sure why we had been given the chemotherapy tablets at the time, but we decided that maybe it was best to take them just in case and it was after all only a short course.

The cancer did not settle down — in fact on our return from Mexico it continued to become more active. The cost of the treatment protocol and the stay in the clinic included a return visit, but for Joe this treatment seemed to have aggravated his cancer and so we did not return for our free visit. As I said, some things work for some people and not for others.

Having now had the time to reminisce on the clinics which we visited my thoughts are that some of the more invasive alternative treatments can sometimes cause an extreme flare in a cancer. This may be the reason why many of these clinics carry out their alternative treatments in conjunction with conventional drugs so that, when the flare occurs, the conventional drugs can be administered when the cancer cells are more sensitized and susceptible to attack.

The Paracelsus Clinic

We had just one visit to The Paracelsus Clinic, Lustmühle, Switzerland, which was on 27th April 2009. I had spoken to the doctor who would be supervising Joe's treatment prior to the visit and he had suggested that Joe's cancer may have already progressed too far for their treatments to be effective. He was honest and, hearing the full details of Joe's current condition, made no promises to be able to help. I told him that I had already tried many different treatments and that Joe was on a good diet with many supplements and alkalising green drinks. We decided to go for two weeks in any case as Dr Seeger spoke so highly about it, despite the fact that Professor Oliver had advised that, in his experience, a patient generally reacts better to treatment when it is administered at home or in his/her own country. We ignored the advice and decided that anything was worth a try. So we travelled there and stayed at the clinic for about ten days. What made us think that it was worth the trip? Take a look at their website _www.paracelsus.ch/paracelsus/paracelsuse/portrait-en/welcome_ which explains in great detail how patients are treated.

Joe's PSA was on the rise again. We wanted to try and do something quickly so arranging the visit to tie in with other commitments was difficult. Unfortunately, Joe had to travel alone and be at the clinic for the first day by himself as I was on a cellular medicine analysis and flow analysis course in Chicago. Joe hated to travel alone and when it came to organising personal things by himself he was completely useless.

We stayed at a hotel in the centre of St Gallen which is a beautiful city in the north east of Switzerland with Lake Constance close by. It is one of the highest cities in Switzerland and has a heavy snowfall in winter. It boasts much history and there are many good restaurants. The clinic was only about ten minute's drive from the hotel.

Joe had an initial appointment with the Patient Counsellor who helps to explain the treatments and supports the patients during their stay. There followed an interview with the doctor who would be recommending Joe's treatment protocol.

Joe had some initial blood tests, a vitamin C infusion and he also had magnet field therapy. There are various different types of magnet field therapy; one method includes the use of static magnets placed on the patient and another involves passing electricity through a coil to create a magnetic field. Some practitioners claim that subjecting certain parts of the body to magneto static fields produced by permanent magnets has beneficial health effects. However, these claims are as yet unproven and no effects on health or healing have been established. Although haemoglobin, the blood protein that carries oxygen, is weakly diamagnetic (creates a magnetic field in opposition to an externally applied magnetic field) and is repulsed by magnetic fields, the magnets used in magnet field therapy are far too weak to have any measurable effect on blood flow.

Joe's first day at the Paracelsus Clinic was uncertain for him as he felt that the treatments here would be no different to the last clinic. Moreover, he was unsettled because I was not with him. People who knew Joe would find this hard to believe, but we rarely show our weaknesses to others do we? Thankfully he agreed to stay after I reassured him that I would be there very soon — I arrived the next day. Once I had seen the doctor to discuss the intended treatment and protocol and was happy that Joe was getting the best treatment, Joe settled down.

Joe had intra-venous (IV) infusions most days which were generally a cocktail of various vitamins, minerals and antioxidants prepared specifically in accordance with the agreed protocol. He had very high doses of intravenous vitamin C. A side–effect of this was that Joe rarely slept during the night if it had been administered in the afternoon. On leaving the clinic we took some of the specially prepared IV preparations home with us, but we could not find anyone to administer them. There was obviously a fear that if anything went wrong that they would be blamed, which was understandable, as they could have been administering anything — even Healthcare at Home couldn't administer it for the same reason.

He had other infusions which were not explained to me. I did ask the nurses what was in the infusions, but they said that they did not know. I thought these to be alkaline infusions and detoxification infusions but in all honesty they could have been anything. I was so adamant about knowing every detail of treatments which were suggested by the NHS and yet here I was allowing treatments to be administered without knowing the full implications. Maybe it was because I believed that the treatments which Joe was having would not kill him because they were not drugs, maybe it was because I believed that there was no further damage that could be done to him because his cancer was at such an advanced stage. A thought that crossed my mind was that maybe it was a miracle infusion specific to the clinic which was going to help Joe's condition so I trusted them. Maybe people who trust the NHS at earlier stages are just more trusting?

Whilst at this clinic Joe also had another treatment which was hyperthermia — local and whole–body.

Hyperthermia

Hyperthermia is a type of treatment that simply mimics a fever by external exposure of special lamps on the body to induce an internal body temperature upwards of 40 degrees centigrade. It is known that heating areas of the body that contain a cancer, or heating the tumour itself, may help to kill cancer cells or make cancer cells more sensitive to the effects of radiation and certain anti–cancer drugs. The procedure is also known to increase blood and lymph circulation, decrease tissue acidity, increase the internal temperature and revitalise the cells, as well as increasing the activity of the immune system locally.

Joe had whole body hyperthermia which involved the whole body being slid into a thermal chamber, like a large incubator or MRI scanner. He had a drip in his arm to receive fluids whilst in the chamber and his heart, blood pressure and temperature were monitored continually. To me it looked frightening, but Joe was completely relaxed in the machine — maybe it reminded him of being in the warmth of the sunshine. I chatted to him whilst he was in the machine and gave him sips of water as his mouth was very dry. Whether this treatment had any beneficial effects I cannot say as Joe felt no change in himself whatsoever.

With local hyperthermia heat is applied to a small area, such as a tumour. Different types of energy may be used to apply heat, including microwave, radiofrequency and ultrasound, dependent upon the type of cancer or tumour. Joe had external applications of local hyperthermia on several occasions. This focused on the lower spine area where Joe had several bony metastatic lesions. Joe did not mind this treatment and did not find it painful.

Many of the alternative cancer clinics are of the opinion that this treatment can be used alongside alternative treatments to boost the immune system. Other clinics believe that it should be used in conjunction with other conventional treatments such as chemotherapy and radiotherapy to make the treatment more effective and the side-effects weaker. The consensus would seem to be that, whichever way it is used, it is an effective treatment.

There is a restaurant at the side of the Paracelsus clinic where the food is extremely tasty, nutritious and healthy, catering mainly for vegetarians. The menus which are offered focus on the most recent findings for the promotion of a hypoallergenic, low carbohydrate and mostly vegetarian diet rich in vegetable oils. The dietician at the clinic discussed our dietary habits with us and provided some additional advice — she also told us about the Coy Diet

Coy Diet

The main focus of the Coy Diet is to block the invasive growth and the metastasis of cancer cells by inhibition of TKTL1 sugar fermentation in cancer cells by activation of a mitochondria based oxidative energy release. Dr Coy discovered the TKTL1 (transketolase-like 1) gene in 1995 when he was working at the German Cancer Center in Heidelberg. Inhibition of the TKTL1 based sugar fermentation leads to an activation of mitochondria facilitating execution of programmed cell death (apoptosis) and induction of reactive oxygen species (ROS) based cell damages. Because of this, the efficacy of natural occurring anti-cancer drugs, as well as standard therapies (chemo- and radiotherapies), can be increased leading to the efficient killing of cancer cells. Therefore, the Coy Diet changes the metabolism of cancer cells from a fermentative metabolism to an oxidative metabolism rendering them sensitive for cancer treatments and blocking metastasis. One important aspect of the Coy Diet is a restriction of carbohydrates (e.g. sugar, starch) leading to the production of ketone bodies (produced by the liver and used as an energy source when glucose is not available) as a tool to monitor oxidative metabolism. To facilitate the metabolic targeting of tumour cells, Dr Coy has developed a special range of products to attempt to make the diet more convenient. These include special protein bread, pasta, lactic acid drinks, jam and chocolate.

The Coy diet products are split into three basic categories;-

- Special oils rich in Omega-3 fatty acids and medium chain triglycerides and tocotrienol which inhibit the glucose fermentation in TKTL1 positive cancer cells
- Lactic acid rich drink which removes the lactic acid from

around the cancer cells

- Special food products rich in proteins and phytochemicals like polyphenols (e.g. quercetin) which inhibit the TKTL1 sugar fermentation in cancer cells

Basically the end result should be that the body's defence cells can attack the cancer cells once the lactic acid shield is removed and stop the cancer cells from multiplying.

The products are only available from Tavarlin in Germany. *www.tavarlin.de/*
Included with kind permission from Johannes F. Coy

Joe had various blood tests at the clinic and the results indicated that the Coy Diet could be beneficial for him. We received the results after we had left the clinic and could not, therefore, get the products for the diet from there. So we sent our son on the mission to Germany with empty suitcases to buy the products required for the diet and bring them home. When he arrived in Germany, he had a one hour taxi journey to reach Tavarlin, which is the only place where the products can be bought. He stayed in a local hotel overnight to await the shop opening the following day so that he could buy the necessary products — what a long home delivery!

Unfortunately, Joe did not stick to the diet for very long, not even for one month, which was probably not long enough to give any results. Special diets are very difficult to follow and Joe was not the best at sticking to any diet for long. Results are not evident straight away from a special diet which makes the patient lose hope. I also think that by this time Joe knew that the cancer was going to get him in the end whatever we tried, so I think that he wanted to enjoy as much pleasure from life as he could and food was always a big pleasure for him.

In summary, it is my opinion that the Paracelsus Clinic is a superb clinic and offers many therapies. However, I believe that we came across this clinic too late in our battle against cancer — let's not forget that Joe's cancer was already stage IV (late stage) and had already spread to his bones on diagnosis. Had we found it sooner, and learnt of the different therapies which are available not just here but in general, then we may have been able to prolong Joe's life even longer. I do not think that the alternative treatments and diet were strong enough to beat Joe's cancer, and it seemed that the combination of the varying alternative therapies bombarding the system at once was not beneficial in his case. The cancer was by then at an advanced stage and fought back aggressively. Towards the end of the first week Joe had another flare in his cancer similar to the flare which he had when he visited the alternative medicine clinic in Mexico and he was in agony with pain in his back and hips. I feel sure that, had he needed chemotherapy or radiotherapy at that time, the cancer was active and ready to be attacked. There is a case, therefore, that it did indeed perform as expected by putting the cancer in a vulnerable position.

I did meet a lady at the Paracelsus Clinic who had suffered an aggressive cancer and she was completely in remission. She was so impressed with what the clinic had done for her that she had moved to live very close to it and was still visiting regularly for immune-boosting therapies. As I said, every cancer is different.

Included with kind permission from the Paracelsus Clinic

The Cancer Clinic

From August 2009, the time when Joe had his first intra–venous chemotherapy, our battle was constant and in January 2010 Joe's health became increasingly worse. He was unable to walk very far without being out of breath and we knew that the time had come to try something else.

There were many clinics from which to choose to go for treatment — the difficulty was choosing the best one for Joe's stage of cancer. We knew that alternative treatments were only going to help at this stage — they would not stop the cancer — it was too aggressive.

I recalled that a few years previously we had been on holiday and I was in the middle of unpacking when Joe called for me to watch something on the television. It was a chat show and the guest was discussing her work with cancer and was describing the book which she had written on the subject.

Remembering this and now eager to know more, I ordered her book. Almost as soon as the book left the postman's hands I began to read. I felt that God was looking down on me and helping me, seeing that I did not know what to do next. Why else would I have remembered this programme, this book, all these years later? As I read, I believed that it held the answers to my questions, shining a light to lead me in the right direction. The book described the different clinics and the treatments which they offered, one of them being the Cancer Clinic (an alias). In my hunger for answers I read the book in a day, having only ever read a handful of books in my life, and within a month we were on our way.

We stayed at a hotel not far from the clinic for three weeks. By the end of our stay it felt like home. We had a very comfortable suite with a kitchen so that we could cook for ourselves. The local supermarket was well-stocked with organic, fresh fruit and vegetables. It would have been impractical to eat in restaurants every day as sometimes Joe was so tired that he just wanted to go back to the room and watch TV or a movie. The hotel staff were fabulous, very attentive, and there was a limousine service which we could have used to take us to the Cancer Clinic every day, but Joe preferred to have our own car. There was a beautiful garden where Joe would often sit in the sun and read.

We arrived at the Cancer Clinic, an impressive glass-fronted structure, on the 17th March 2010. The reception area was small and welcoming, quite different to the façade. Joe was by now very weak and still unable to walk far without being out of breath — he definitely could not have climbed a flight of stairs when we arrived.

We immediately felt that the staff were friendly and went out of their way to make us feel at ease. We firstly had a meeting with our Doctor, Dr Jacobs (an alias), an extremely compassionate and caring woman in addition to being a brilliant professional. She was our main point of contact at the clinic and dealt with all matters swiftly and efficiently. We also met with the Director and Founder of the Clinic, Dr Fredericks (an alias), a very down to earth man who explained to us in layman's terms how the treatment worked. The theories and treatments practiced are considered by some as highly contentious but the focus has been on 'personalised' care long before it became an established focus of modern research. Our experience of the Cancer Clinic was one which we felt was of benefit. Considering Joe's late stage of cancer, all orthodox treatments had failed and we were willing to try anything, even if considered by some to be ineffective.

On the first day various blood samples were taken to test for, amongst other things, over-expression of genetic markers (basically to see if there is any predisposition in the DNA to cancer or other diseases depending upon the tests being carried out). Joe also had a general health examination.

The results of the blood tests revealed elevations of HER2 (human epidermal growth factor receptor), basically a protein associated with a poor prognosis in prostate cancer when elevated, and elevation of VEGF (vascular endothelial growth factor), an indicator for prostate cancer. He was noted to have a **CTC** (circulating tumour cells) count of 296 cell/7.5ml of blood. I don't know if this is a large number or not, but seeing that number in such a small sample was a shock knowing that each one had the potential to plant itself somewhere else and grow a new tumour. I never really let myself think any further than the actual facts i.e. it was in Joe's bones, never realising that obviously if it was in his bones it was in his blood too. But somehow bones didn't seem as bad because bones are static and isolated, but blood is everywhere which makes the reality of the situation much worse. Due to his elevated genetic markers and CTCs he was started on various different treatments which would not have been available for him to try in England.

On the second day Joe was sent for a **PET scan** of the whole body. My research suggests that this would appear to be one of the safest and most accurate scans available as it delivers the lowest levels of radiation. When the results were ready the radiologist showed the scans to me. It was frightening to see the extent and activity of the cancer. I never made Joe aware of how active the cancer was.

On the third day Joe began a course of Amino Care A10 supplements. Amino Care A10 is a mixture of amino acids, an amino acid derivative and vitamin B2. It supports the defence system of the body and contributes to the regulation of normal cell division.

Joe began **bevacizumab** on the 23rd March 2010. This would not have been available to him in England. It was not used at that time for prostate cancer but it did have very favourable results. It was administered every two weeks. This was the popular breast cancer drug that everyone was fighting for and was difficult to come by as it is costly. He was also given **lapatinib** and **rilutek**. Along with this medication he was also having diethylstilbestrol, dexamethasone, degarelix and zoledronic acid, plus his alternative supplements.

We drove to the clinic every day for a medical assessment and for any new treatments. Joe was a brilliant driver who compared himself to a homing pigeon. It was true — once he had been somewhere he would always be able to find it again. Unbelievably, on the third day he could not find his way to the clinic. We drove around and around, up and down the freeway. I was afraid to drive on the freeway with its six lanes and very fast traffic. Nevertheless I eventually had no option but to take the wheel. Incredibly I went directly to the clinic without a problem. I could see that Joe was tired and confused. To see him so was difficult as he was an incredibly strong, vibrant man, always in control and would never express his misery or pain. Gosh, I wish that I could have kept him alive.

Initially Joe's body tolerated all of the drugs well. The only problem which he had was that his feet were a little sore and the skin on them became red and very dry, a known side–effect of lapatinib. I would apply cream (udderly cream which is a greaseless, stainless moisturising cream which is especially effective on dry areas caused by chemotherapy) twice a day which helped the condition. In less than one week of taking the new medication, Joe was feeling and looking better than he had for some time. He was no longer out of breath — he even came to the gym with me! He was no longer confused, insisting on driving backwards and forwards to the clinic even though he had been advised that he shouldn't.

The dietician at the clinic provided advice on a healthy diet but, because I had already changed our diet so much, the only suggestion was to compensate for Joe's potassium levels being very low, which is a problem even for healthy people due to the effects that low levels can have on the kidneys, so she recommended that he eat more beans and gave him a list of potassium rich foods to increase in his diet. She also recommended no dairy, no meat, a mainly vegetarian diet and more fluids — Joe never drank much water.

At the end of the three weeks we left the clinic armed with the medication and with Joe feeling very much better than when we had arrived, so all in all a successful visit.

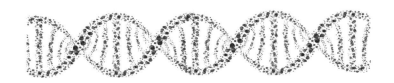

9 — Osteonecrosis of the Jaw

When we returned home from the Cancer Clinic Joe was settling down well with his new treatments. Orally he was taking lapatinib, rilutek, **sorafenib** and bevacizumab.

By this time Joe was basically back to his old self and was feeling great. I was so happy and relieved as I had felt that I was losing him. His CTCs had reduced by 100 when we left, so he was also happy. The cancer was extremely widespread in his bones at this stage — there were too many lesions to count, but still there was no evidence to show any spread to the soft tissue or organs. In the medical discharge summary it stated 'the patient's condition currently is satisfactory; however the prognosis remains guarded'.

Not long after our return home Joe was in extreme pain from a swelling around his tooth. He went to the dentist who advised that Joe must firstly have a course of antibiotics to destroy the infection before he could decide whether to remove the tooth or not. The pain did not go away and became progressively worse and finally on April 18th 2010 there was no option but to seek medical attention at the hospital as Joe was in agony and the antibiotics were having no effect.

Whether it was the medical staff's unfamiliarity with a cancer case such as Joe's, whether it was overwork which meant that they didn't have the patience for a difficult case, whether because we had been so used to the care which we had been receiving at the Cancer Clinic, where time and individual attention were not in scarce supply which made this situation seem worse, I don't know. But what I do know, in my opinion, is that the staff were not compassionate, not understanding of the predicament in which we found ourselves and not interested in understanding the detail which, as it turned out, was a big mistake. Whatever the reasons, it took an unreasonable amount of time for them to accept the severity of the situation, but eventually they listened and it was decided that Joe would have the tooth extracted at the dental Hospital the following morning. He was also given different and stronger antibiotics as we were advised that the current tablets were not the most effective for his condition. He was given metronidazole and amoxicillin, both common antibiotics.

We returned to the dental hospital the following morning. I was not allowed in and Joe had to go in alone. I waited nervously for over an hour, knowing that he would be anxious without me to ask the right questions for him if needed. Apparently, a student was doing the procedure and when Joe came out she had not as yet even removed the tooth. The decaying tooth was attached to a bridge, and all that she had done was to cut through the bridge to separate the teeth. In doing so she had cut into the gum causing it to bleed and become extremely sore. The intention was that he would go back after lunch to have the tooth extracted by this student. I had a gut feeling that something was not quite right, sensations which had developed over time as I had become intimate with Joe's cancer, and so we did not go back. Instead I called my dentist, who is also a surgeon, and explained the situation to him. He arranged for Joe to visit him the following day. That evening, where the incision had been made, copious amounts of horrific smelling puss oozed out. It stank! The pain was becoming much less as the infectious puss left his mouth. Joe squeezed and squeezed at it until there was no more and the relief from pain on his face was obvious. We never really gave much thought to what had caused the puss, which was probably an abscess, as the severity of the impending tooth problem was about to engulf us. Joe went to see my dentist the following day. He apologised that he could not pull the tooth out as Joe was taking bisphosphonates, which are routinely used to treat bone metastasis, but are known to have the potential side–effect of osteonecrosis of the jaw. (Osteonecrosis of the bones occurs when bones lose their blood supply. The bones eventually die and can collapse. Cancer patients are a high risk group for this disease.) He therefore recommended that the best course of action would be a root canal filling and cleaning of the tooth.

At this stage we knew nothing of osteonecrosis of the jaw. Joe returned for the tooth procedure. The dentist, the highly trained assistant of my dentist, was very gentle and professional. He cleaned out the canals of the tooth, leaving a disinfectant solution inside it for a while to ensure that all of the bacteria had been removed before finishing the procedure. Joe went back in to the dentist to have the procedure completed, and when the dentist looked in his mouth he was extremely shocked by what he saw. I knew that something was wrong because the dentist went sheet white. Apparently he had never before witnessed osteonecrosis of the jaw and he was horrified. He called for my dentist who confirmed that his diagnosis was indeed correct. He was afraid to do any further work on Joe at that point as it was as if part of his jaw had disappeared and you could see inside him! It was horrendous — I can think of no other word to describe it.

My dentist recommended an excellent cranio–maxillofacial specialist surgeon who practiced in London. Such specialists treat diseases, defects and injuries relating to the face, head and neck and also the mouth and jaw. I researched the problem on the internet before the appointment. My findings were that there was little that could be done. Apparently this was something relatively new in the medical world. The indications were that it is generally the result of having dentistry work done whilst taking, or having taken, bisphosphonates, which Joe had taken in the form of zoledronic acid. The only positive information which I was able to find was that taking ciprofloxacin (used to treat bacterial infections) and metronidazole (an anti–infection agent) twice daily could control the osteonecrosis. The specialist, who was an extremely considerate, understanding, professional gentleman, agreed with my findings. He X–rayed Joe's jaw and requested that Professor Oliver arrange a scan to rule out any cancer spread to the area, which subsequently turned out to be negative. The specialist prescribed the ciprofloxacin and metronidazole long term. A word of warning — it was extremely difficult to obtain these from the GP for periods in excess of two months even though we travelled frequently and it caused problems getting back to the GP each time for a repeat prescription, even with a private prescription. But I never gave up and always managed to get the tablets. The specialist recommended another top surgeon in London who performed operations to help osteonecrosis. Unfortunately, due to Joe's state of health, there was nothing that he could do or recommend to help us.

Joe had been taking zoledronic acid intravenously every month. Zoledronic acid is meant to strengthen the bones and it is said to help reduce the spread of secondary cancer in the bones. It was of great benefit, but the possible side–effect, osteonecrosis of the jaw, was very hard to live with. We were never made aware of this side-effect when Joe was prescribed zoledronic acid. I think that, before deciding to take this drug, there must be certainty that there are no known dental issues, bridges, root canals or fillings. That is not to say that these could not develop after beginning the treatment, as with Joe, but at least it narrows the odds.

Joe could not eat certain foods as he could not chew properly and certain foods would get inside the hole. It was recommended that he eat only soft foods, liquid drinks and vegetable drinks. This was all that he could take as nourishment until he died. In severe cases, osteonecrosis of the jaw can actually cause the jaw to break off. The thought of this terrified Joe. This problem caused him an immense amount of pain. He described the osteonecrosis as the worst side-effect of all of the drugs and it was a continual problem that required constant supervision — I had a small torch with which to inspect it on a daily basis.

This was the start of a roller coaster of good and bad days, highs and lows and the downward spiral to Joe's terrible health and the end of our fight. Professor Oliver at one stage suggested some radiotherapy to Joe's jaw to try and ease the pain, but this could be detrimental with osteonecrosis, so apart from the long-term antibiotics and the continuous use of pain killers there was nothing much that we could do.

There was a hospital which was using immune system stimulation treatments which I thought might help Joe. However, Dr Jacobs advised that immune system stimulants would produce additional problems in that his body would try to stimulate recovery from osteonecrosis and any additional stimulation might lead to the production of antibodies against other tissues of his body. All in all it would mean a massive and constant strain on the immune system and so definitely not a suitable course of treatment at that time. Dr Jacobs was extremely upset when she got the news that Joe had osteonecrosis of the jaw. She was perfectly aware that the symptoms would be severely distressing for Joe, and painful, and that his overall well-being would be affected as his immune system would have to work overtime just to cope with this, never mind coping with treatments and cancer.

Since we had left the Cancer Clinic, Dr Jacobs had always been available for help and advice. The follow-up support service which the clinic provided was excellent. Dr Jacobs requested that I find a place where the CTCs could be tested in England. This proved to be very difficult to find but I eventually came across Source Bioscience in Nottingham (*www.sourcebioscience.com*) who were able to perform the CTC blood tests. They were extremely helpful. They were also able to test the HER2 and VEGF genetic markers.

Joe continued to do well on his treatment protocol, but his jaw continued to cause increasing pain and eventually, at the end of June 2010, Professor Oliver was forced to prescribe oral morphine for it which was effective.

Joe had a period towards the end of June 2010 when all of the tablets were making him sick and he could not eat as he had no appetite whatsoever. He would only have liquid intake. Dr Jacobs gave him a break from the tablets and the GP prescribed metoclopramide (commonly used to treat sickness and nausea) which helped a great deal. Joe was soon eating better, stopped being sick and was able to restart all of his tablets. At the beginning of July 2010 he resumed treatment with bevacizumab. At the end of July Dr Jacobs became concerned about Joe's PSA which was rising again. I had also received the results for the genetic markers HER2 which were still showing elevation and also VEGF was still high. Docetaxel chemotherapy was added to attempt to combat this and the combination worked well. Dr Jacobs also wanted to replace sorafenib with pazopanib, which slows the growth of cancer cells, as she felt that it would provide better overall results, and this was Fed-exed to us without delay.

The treatment plan worked well, but throughout the pain in Joe's jaw never really settled. Some days Joe was in agony and would not take any of his medication. This jaw problem was most definitely proving to be the worst thing that could possibly have happened. Joe had to take dexamethasone corticosteroid (a steroid) on a daily basis, which seemed to help to keep the jaw pain under some control. I would alter the daily dose according to Joe's pain needs. When Joe had a flare with the cancer I would have to increase the steroid dose, in accordance with Professor Oliver's guidelines, to sometimes as much as 12mg and then gradually decrease it over the following days until the pain was under control. It was a real case of trial and error with the aim of reducing the steroids to the lowest level possible. The steroids would make Joe puff up all over, especially his face, and they would sometimes make him a little aggressive — not good for a man in pain and distressed already.

It is easy to try to find blame for someone being in pain. So who was to blame for Joe's jaw pain, which turned out to be the worst thing that he had to face as far as a detrimental effect on his quality of life was concerned? It was negligent of the NHS hospital staff who recommended removal of his tooth before checking whether Joe was taking bisphosphonates. Why was a student operating on such a sick man and why did she cut through the skin when separating the bridge before she was going to remove the tooth? No–one warned us about the possible dangers of osteonecrosis of the jaw when the zoledronic acid was prescribed. Too late to throw stones — but a warning to be aware not to blindly trust medical staff who may not always know best. I kept a diary throughout Joe's illness detailing the drugs which he had been prescribed and when they were prescribed. With hindsight, I would have given this to any new person examining Joe and would have insisted that they examine it — then they could not say that they had not been told about a particular treatment or problem and would be responsible should a bad turn of events occur, so they might be more diligent.

In October 2010 Joe developed a lump in his jaw at the osteonecrosis site and his PSA was again rising. He was also sleeping a lot. He was becoming gradually weaker from all of the treatments and Professor Oliver believed that Joe would benefit from a break from the treatment so that we could reintroduce it again in one month's time before we went on our Christmas break. But at the same time Dr Jacobs was keen to start Joe on two other treatments to slow down the activity in his bones, namely **teriparatide** injection (used to treat osteoporosis and prevent bone loss) and denosumab (inhibits a protein which signals bone removal). Professor Oliver refused to agree to these to begin with.

The Cancer Clinic wanted Joe to have another PET scan, which he did on the 8th November 2010. The results of the scan were not good and showed widespread activity in most of his bones. There was also an area of abnormal soft tissue activity immediately below the right lower jaw associated with some soft tissue swelling of approximately 1.17cm diameter. Having reviewed the scans, Dr Fredericks felt that Joe was no longer suffering from adenocarcinoma (cancer focused around the prostate gland), and that his disease had transformed into neuroendocrine (highly indifferentiated and evidenced in other organs) cancer. He believed that this was the reason for the progression picked up by the scan together with falling PSA, as this type of cancer does not produce PSA. Dr Fredericks proposed that, to address the neuroendocrine features and reverse the disease process, the treatment plan must change so the drugs listed in Appendix 9 were suggested (very specific to Joe's case and stage of cancer so included for completeness only).

With the amazing help of all of our medical experts, we managed to obtain all of the new drugs, with the exception of **vorinostat** which the Cancer Clinic arranged to Fed-ex to us immediately hence negating the need for us to travel to Houston. He began the new treatment protocol on Monday 22nd November 2010. Joe made a great improvement immediately. He was no longer sleeping all day and was again much more focused. The only problem was that he was not eating much and was losing weight.

Professor Oliver finally agreed on teriparatide to help re-grow the bone in Joe's jaw, strengthen his bones and slow the cancer activity in his bones. On the 3rd December 2010 the vorinostat arrived and I immediately administered it to Joe. However, the same evening Joe became very hot, his blood pressure started to rise and his leg and foot became very swollen. Joe was admitted to hospital and found to be suffering from deep vein thrombosis.

Following the deep vein thrombosis, Joe had to have an enoxaparin sodium (Clexane, Lovenox, Xaparin) injection (blood thinning injection) daily, which I had to administer. He also carried on taking all of his tablets over the Christmas period, except for the vorinostat and the bortezomib injection, which we hoped to reintroduce after Christmas, but he was very weak. Continually stopping and starting treatments due to complications did affect the true benefits.

In summary, the Cancer Clinic can prove to be very expensive for many budgets, but even at Joe's late stage it gave him an extra ten months of life of which six months was quality life. Had Joe not developed the osteonecrosis of the jaw and the deep vein thrombosis, which were both side-effects from the drugs, he would have gone on a lot longer I am sure. So, for us, finding the Cancer Clinic and receiving the support which they provided was worth its weight in gold.

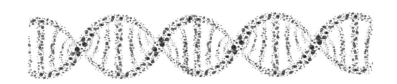

10 — Lifestyle Changes and Known Risk Factors

Following the diagnosis we tried various alternative treatments to support Joe's health and to help to control the cancer, and we knew that we must make lifestyle changes to ensure that we did everything possible to succeed. Here I explain the many changes which we made and how we managed to achieve three years with no conventional treatment and prolong Joe's life.

Stress

It is well documented that the effects of prolonged stress can be detrimental to health and that the body can react in various ways, even succumbing to serious illness. Stress wears down the body's immune system so that when disease or illness attacks, the body is too tired to deal with it or defend itself. Stress itself can cause digestive, fertility and urinary problems as well as depleting the immune system, thereby increasing the likelihood of suffering from colds, flu, headaches, sleeplessness, depression and anxiety. These symptoms can then increase and create a whole new list of issues for the body to deal with. Although stress in itself does not cause cancer, the depleted state of the body can make it more difficult for any defence against cancer to be raised. Also, the symptoms of stress can cause people to turn to excessive alcohol consumption, smoking, lack of exercise or over–eating which *can* increase the risks of cancer.

Research shows that people under stress do not respond to treatment as well as people who are not stressed. There are various methods available to help to reduce stress: yoga, exercise, walking, counselling, change of job and medication to name but a few.

Although I tried to steer Joe towards a less stressful existence, I must admit that I was largely unsuccessful. Having said that, Joe was a man who thrived on stress, being constantly on the go and constantly problem–solving, so for him I believe that if he had relaxed he may have lost much of his fight to live.

Joe was a businessman and, like all businessmen, stress comes as part of the package. He would say that there was no point in worrying, yet he would spend sleepless nights mulling over solutions to problems. But the stress never appeared to be a problem and his behaviour around his family and friends would never show signs of stress. He could lose his temper like the rest of us, but not in an irrational way and not excessively.

I saw the change in Joe over a period of time as the cancer progressed. He would always deny that he was stressed, but the change in his behaviour betrayed the truth. He would become irritable, angering easily when people made mistakes or did not follow instructions, which was not the professional manner in which he usually conducted himself. His patience grew thin, even with me, and sometimes it was hard to see these as symptoms of stress and forgive them. He would have odd days when he would totally ignore all of our hard work at achieving a healthy lifestyle, eating excessively to the point of feeling ill, and likewise with drink, but thankfully these incidents were intermittent and short–lived. He would often be silent and deep in thought, but if I questioned him he would say that he was no different and that he had learnt to be silent in solitary confinement all those years ago in prison — but I knew that he was different. In addition to his business stresses, which he had always coped with without showing any symptoms, I have no doubt that the stress of fighting his cancer and the worry of whether or not he would survive constantly hung over him and were too large a burden. So, despite his denials, I know that he was suffering from stress, and I could do nothing about it. This was heartbreaking because I knew that this was hindering our progress visibly.

So if I failed so miserably why have I included this here? Because I tried everything that I could to help him, but the only person who could help him was himself, yet the catalyst of the threat of death was just too strong for him to overcome. He refused to talk to anyone about his stress, his feelings, his obvious pent–up frustrations, but I believe that this would have helped him and helped our fight. So, for this reason, I have included this, because I wish with all my heart that I could have encouraged him to have had more than just two visits to alternative healing therapists (who treat the mind as well as the body), where he opened up and told them how he felt, which must have helped. Counselling is also a weapon (not one that Joe or I would ever have considered due to our lack of experience with it) and can help to reduce anxiety and stress, thereby strengthening the immune system so that it is better able to fend off disease — including cancer.

Exercise

There is much research to suggest that the likelihood of developing certain cancers is significantly reduced in people who undertake regular exercise, and that physically active people are less likely to suffer from mild depression and stay mentally alert as they age. Indeed, regular exercise has many health benefits. It has long been established as fact that increased physical exercise has beneficial effects on various conditions such as osteoarthritis, cardiovascular disease, respiratory diseases, cancer, diabetes, osteoporosis and obesity.

There is no need to run marathons or push your body to the limits in any type of exercise — it is meant to be enjoyable, with little and often being equally beneficial. Just ten minutes of moderate exercise is enough to improve mood, vigour and also decrease fatigue. However, to obtain all of the benefits from exercise, not just the mood–improving aspects, thirty minutes of moderate exercise every day is recommended — though not so easy to achieve! Moderate intensity aerobic activity is the initial aim, working hard enough to raise your heart rate and break into a sweat. Examples of moderate intensity aerobic activities are: walking fast, water aerobics, riding a bike on level ground or with a few hills, playing doubles tennis, even pushing a lawnmower. Sometimes it's hard to find the get up and go to exercise, but afterwards the benefits of the good endorphins flowing around the body are immediately felt and mood and spirit are lifted. This is because exercise decreases the stress hormones such as cortisol (which suppresses the immune system) and endorphins are released. Endorphins are the body's natural feel–good chemicals, and when they are released your mood is boosted naturally. Endorphins are defined as hormone-like substances which are produced in the brain and function as the body's natural painkillers during exercise, being so powerful that they actually mask pain. As well as endorphins, exercise also releases adrenaline, serotonin, and dopamine which all promote feelings of well–being.

Although Joe was always on the go he did not exercise regularly because he found it quite boring, so one of the first steps for him was to join a gym. When he was diagnosed he realised that exercise was an important aspect of ensuring that his body was strong enough to fight the cancer, so he ignored his boredom and used his willpower to work–out and take part in aerobic exercise — we also cycled and swam which he enjoyed. Joe's mood was always better when he was exercising. He would pat his tummy when he came back from the gym and say, 'you see, I am losing weight already. Soon I will be a shadow of my former self'. The exercise also encouraged him to have better eating habits as he felt better in himself.

Recently I struck up a conversation with a gentleman on the train. Having noticed my papers on health and diet, he asked whether I was a nutritionist. I explained that I was writing a book, promised to my late husband, a book to share our experiences in fighting cancer and hopefully help others reduce the risk of developing the disease. The man, let's call him Andrew, had lost his father at forty–three years of age to bowel cancer. We discussed how Andrew's father had always worked long hours, was constantly stressed and never found much time for relaxation, or for exercise. After talking with Andrew, who explained how he was perhaps going through that same stage in his life — no time for himself, no time for exercise, eating badly — he thanked me and said that I had given him the wake–up call that he needed. He assured me that he would definitely buy my book and would now begin to take better care of his well–being. He explained that his wife had bought a dog and that he was on his way home, back to Birmingham, after working all week in Yorkshire, to meet him. He was excited that, as a start, he could walk the dog, get exercise, fresh air and relaxation. He would also start to play golf, he decided. Golf is a great sport for most, offering relaxation, beautiful scenery, moderate exercise, fresh air — and if you are lucky a dose of sunshine which we all need. Hopefully, Andrew will have made those lifestyle changes and change the course of his life. Is it about time that you did the same?

Eating Habit Changes

There has been much public awareness in recent years about the foods which are bad for the health — processed foods, takeaways, sweet foods — and these were immediately eliminated from Joe's diet. He adopted a mainly vegetarian diet accompanied by fish, with meat once a week as a treat. I would always buy wild or line–caught fish, not farmed, and organic meat whenever possible. A large part of Joe's diet was fresh fruit, vegetables and salads. He would use extra virgin organic olive oil as a dressing with some organic herbs and sea salt. He loved fruit so much, especially peaches and nectarines, but unfortunately I had to hide the fruit bowl from him as he could eat as many as six peaches one after another.

Fruit is good for you, but only in moderation as it contains much natural fruit sugar, and sugar is the favourite food of cancer. I ensured that Joe only ate fruit in the morning as it requires specific enzymes to break it down and, as the day goes on, the enzymes which break down fruit aren't produced as efficiently as earlier in the day. I also never allowed him to eat fruit after a meal because, if the digestive system is already dealing with food from the main meal, the fruit has to wait for the different enzymes so that it can be digested and begins to ferment in the gut, which is not good for the body. It is ironic that given a choice between the fruit bowl and a sticky dessert that the sticky dessert would actually be the best choice from a digestive perspective, although obviously not from a calorific perspective. Decisions, decisions.

I constantly searched for new diets, new supplements, and whenever I found something which I felt would benefit our fight, I would change Joe's eating habits accordingly. Joe tried a raw food diet for a while, but this was never going to be a long–term solution — it was monotonous and time–consuming to prepare so not very practical either. I would juice fresh, organic fruit in the morning and vegetable juice through the day and Joe would snack on raw vegetables. I did, however, continue to prepare fresh fruit juices when Joe fancied them which were an inducement to drink some less appealing vegetable juices which didn't have the sweetness. I found a very efficient juicer which was simple to use and, above all, easy to clean called Vitalmax Oscar 900 (widely available on the internet). We also used to have 'green days' when together we would eat only vegetables which were green — these have anti–inflammatory and antioxidant properties.

I read a book over twenty years ago on weight loss and food combining and, since it made perfect sense to me, I have tried to put the ideologies explained in the book to use on myself ever since. Wrongly combining foods i.e. eating different categories of food together on the same plate, can lead to putrefaction and fermentation of the food leading to acid indigestion, flatulence, heartburn and, even worse, poor nutrition. In turn, this can lead to toxic acids being produced, poor detoxification and low energy. Adopting this method of eating can eliminate feelings of bloating, discomfort and fatigue following a meal.

The basic idea is that proteins and carbohydrates should not be eaten together. Examples of bad combinations would be fish and chips (protein and carbohydrate), meat and potatoes (protein and carbohydrate), cheese and bread (protein/fat and carbohydrate), and egg with toast (protein and carbohydrate). The digestion of food takes up energy and the digestion of foods requiring various different digestive enzymes drains the body of energy for other activities. For cancer sufferers, food combining is crucial as the body and the immune system are already weakened and lacking in energy and need food which is nutritious and easy to digest. The downside is that, at a time when the patient is struggling with so many assaults on the body and mind, this is quite a disciplined way of eating and potentially removes one more enjoyable element of living. Nevertheless, the benefits of following this eating methodology provide immediate results.

Other nutritionists e.g. sports nutritionists, may have a different view, as for sports men and women the body has other requirements from their food. There are also various illnesses which require specific nutrition from their food intake and this diet may not be appropriate for them, but for a cancer patient food combining is, I believe, a must. The body is already under pressure to function efficiently whilst fighting the cancer and consequently needs to obtain maximum nutritional value from every mouthful of food, utilising as little energy as possible to process it. However, as I have said before, I would always recommend discussing with your medical practitioner any intended changes to your diet or treatments before going ahead.

Organic Foods

A change to mainly organic foods was another of the lifestyle changes which we made, ensuring that wherever possible all of our fruit and vegetables were organic. Organic farming recognises the connection between our health and how the food which we eat is produced. Artificial fertilisers and pesticides are banned and farmers develop fertile soil by rotating crops and using compost, manure and clover. Under organic standards genetically modified (GM) crops and ingredients are banned. Some fruit and vegetables are safe to eat without necessarily being organic, but some are highly contaminated with pesticides. Although the full impact of the effect of pesticides on the human body and the environment is not known, they have been linked to various diseases, lowered IQ and a higher incidence of ADHD in children. Basically, if you feed your body too much fat, additives, chemicals and toxins, they cannot be properly disposed of. The result is that your body stores these toxins, poisons and fats until it can get rid of them. It is also important to note that as well as spraying the produce with pesticides to produce attractive fruit and vegetables, some food manufacturers often inject the foods which they sell with chemicals in order to prolong their 'shelf life' and to maintain a fresh and appealing appearance. Farmers also inject hormones into their crops to boost the volume of their harvest, so eating these crops might not be as healthy as you think. By exclusively eating organic food you can seriously limit the number of toxins which are being introduced into your body which will ease the burden on overworked body systems.

There has been much research regarding organic food and whether or not it is actually better for you. Several reports have stated categorically that there are definite benefits, whilst other studies have asserted that the only definite benefit is that there is obviously reduced exposure to toxins from pesticides. There remains a consensus that no official body will state that there is any nutritional benefit from consuming organically produced foods. The same consensus refuses to state that GM foods can be harmful. GM food production remains a major industry and a move to organic food production would hurt this industry badly. You may draw your own conclusions.

There is a guide called EWG's (Environmental Working Group) shopper's guide, _(www.ewg.org)._ This guide provides details of the 'dirty dozen' and the 'clean fifteen'. The dirty dozen are the dozen basic fruits and vegetables which should be bought as organic as a priority as these were found to have the highest pesticide residues. The twelve most contaminated fruits and vegetables described generally as the 'dirty dozen' are:

- Apples
- Celery
- Sweet bell peppers
- Peaches
- Strawberries
- Nectarines
- Grapes
- Spinach
- Lettuce
- Cucumbers
- Blueberries
- Potatoes

Plus Green beans, kale/collard greens.

Green beans and collard greens did not meet traditional dirty dozen criteria but were commonly contaminated with highly toxic organophosphate insecticides. These insecticides are toxic to the nervous system and have been largely removed from agriculture over the past decade. However, they are not banned and still show up on some food crops. Number one on the list is the apple. According to data, the average conventionally grown apple has more pesticide on it than any other fruit or vegetable.

According to the Environment Working Group's analysis of USDA (U.S. Department of Agriculture) data, pesticides showed up on ninety–eight percent of the more than seven hundred apple samples tested (yes, they were washed), and it wasn't just one pesticide either — apples from around the country, domestically grown and imported, were found to have up to forty–eight different kinds of pesticides on them.

Now we come to the 'clean fifteen'. These are the fifteen fruits and vegetables which, according to the EWG, contain the lowest pesticide residue:

- Onions
- Sweetcorn
- Pineapples
- Avocado
- Cabbage
- Sweet Peas
- Asparagus
- Mangoes
- Eggplant
- Kiwi
- Cantaloupe Melon
- Sweet Potatoes
- Grapefruit
- Watermelon
- Mushrooms

Copyright © Environmental Working Group, www.ewg.org. Reprinted with permission

Although mushrooms and sweetcorn are on the 'clean fifteen' list, Joe and I never ate these two foods.

Mushrooms all contain amounts of the mycotoxin amanitin which, in large amounts, will kill a human almost instantly. Mycotoxins are naturally occurring chemicals which are produced by specific moulds. They can grow on a variety of different crops and foodstuffs including cereals, nuts, spices, dried fruits and coffee, usually in warm and humid conditions. Although the amount of mycotoxins in mushrooms may in some cases be negligible, it nonetheless has the ability to cause adverse health conditions in humans. Certain mycotoxins can cause damage to DNA and cause cancer in animal species. There is also evidence that they can cause liver cancer in humans. Other mycotoxins have various ill effects on health including kidney damage, stomach problems, reproductive disorders or suppression of the immune system. There are statutory levels of a range of mycotoxins permitted in food and animal feed set out by European directives and Commission regulations, an estimate of the tolerable daily intake of mycotoxin which someone can be exposed to daily over a lifetime without it posing a significant risk to health, but surely this isn't a good thing that this restriction is required and should be warning enough not to eat mushrooms.

If corn is harvested and stored in good conditions, then the risks of the mycotoxin fungus developing are drastically reduced. However, if the corn is stored in a humid or hot environment, then this encourages the incubation of the mycotoxins. It is impossible for a person eating corn to tell how the corn has been stored and whether or not it contains mycotoxins.

Tomatoes

There have been multiple studies on lycopene consumption. Lycopene is an antioxidant compound and tomatoes provide substantial amounts. There is much evidence to suggest that Lycopene provides protection against cancers of the lung, stomach and prostate and it has been shown to inhibit cancer cell growth. Joe ate large amounts of tomatoes and tomato sauces after his diagnosis.

Manuka Honey

We replaced sugar with Manuka honey for sweetening. Sugar is not good as it is a friend of cancers. But what makes Manuka honey different to other honey? Known as the 'healing honey' it comes exclusively from the East Cape region of New Zealand where bees pollinate the Manuka trees. It has a UMF (Unique Manuka Factor) of between 10 and 20. The higher the number, the better and more expensive is the honey. It is very stable and doesn't change when exposed to heat. It has antibacterial properties, kills bad bacteria and relieves the discomfort of skin ulcers, burns and other wounds, so much so that it is used to cover wounds and provide a safe environment in which wounds can heal.

As a sweetener, therefore, it is far superior to sugar which has no benefits except taste.

Soya (Soy) Milk

We changed from cow's milk and only drank soya milk.

Soya milk is produced from soya beans and is available fresh and organic. However, always ensure that there are no nasty additives to the brand which you buy just as with any other product. It takes a little while to get used to the taste but, once converted, the creamier, sweeter, nutty taste is enjoyable. Soya milk is a good source of protein whilst being low in fat and carbohydrates. Soya milk does not contain lactose and is therefore also suitable for the lactose intolerant. The biggest benefit of soya milk is isoflavones. These are chemicals very similar to oestrogen, making it very effective on the effects of the female menopause. Isoflavones are connected to the effective control of many health conditions including certain cancers, heart disease, diabetes and high blood pressure. Soya milk also provides additional heart protection with **phytochemicals** which are found in abundance in soya milk. Phytochemicals are compounds produced by plants and are found in fruit, vegetables, beans, grains and other plants. Some of the more commonly known phytochemicals include beta carotene, ascorbic acid (vitamin C), folic acid and vitamin E. There is evidence to suggest that certain phytochemicals can prevent the formation of **carcinogens** (substances that cause cancer) and help to prevent its spread in the body. Certain phytochemicals have antioxidant properties which are helpful in the fight against cancer.

Water

Good quality water is crucial for optimal health as, without it, the body cannot detoxify itself as it is needed for every process of detoxification. Insufficient water intake leads to the accumulation of toxins and waste in the fat cells, tissues and throughout the body. Over time, the body can no longer deal with this accumulation and the body halts, the result being some form of disease, heart attack or stroke. Just as a plant without water will eventually die, so will the body.

Joe did not drink much water, hence why I encouraged him to drink the greens drink (discussed later) every day. During my research I came across articles on water, becoming increasingly conscious about the water which we drank and where it came from. We used to drink only bottled water as, having read about the potential additives in tap water, I gambled that bottled water could only be better. However, I hadn't realised that the PH content can vary quite dramatically between different brands. If the PH is below 7 then the water is basically acidic — certain bottled waters have a PH of 5 or 6, which means that it is actually doing more harm than good to your body. The PH of the water should be on the bottle for information.

I always chose glass bottles if possible to try to avoid any PCBs from the plastic bottles (PCBs are toxic substances within the plastic which can leak into the liquid, particularly if opened for too long or left in the sunshine or heat). However, PCBs can also be found in tap water along with other contaminants ranging from arsenic, heavy metals, pesticides, herbicides, chemicals, bacteria — the list is endless. Chlorine, a poison designed to kill living organisms which may be present, is added to the water and consequently may be ingested. This begs the question of which is worse, the chlorine or the bugs?

I now have a water ionizer — there are several on the market — which separates out the positive ions from the negative ions within the water. It provides water with a lower PH — suitable for many uses including kitchen cleaning, food preparation, skin conditions and alternative disinfectant — and water with a higher PH — water of optimum quality for drinking and achieving an alkaline balance within the body. I have also attached filters to the system to ensure that all unwanted chemicals are eliminated. If an ionizer is outside of your budget, then purifying PH drops (discussed later), or another form of water filter system such as a BRITA filter can be used.

Foods Etc. Which We Avoided

I feel that it is important to repeat myself and state that the following changes which we made were felt to be appropriate for Joe, and were made following discussion with our medical practitioner. I would never recommend making dietary or treatment changes without such referral. It may be that the type and stage of your cancer or health issue may require a food which was deemed to be unsuitable in Joe's instance but may contain a necessary nutrient for your body. I will now explain the foods and products which we avoided and why.

Red Meat

The fact that red meat consumption increases the risk of chronic diseases including heart disease and cancer is well documented.

A most alarming discovery came during a visit from our local pig farmer. He called to see us in December to ask whether we would like some pork for Christmas as a gift. Although I have not eaten meat for over twenty years and Joe never ate pork, we decided to accept his offer and give the meat as a gift to our friends and family. The pig farmer assured us that he would put a couple of pigs to one side for us and that they would be ready in a few weeks time. Knowing our passion for healthy living, he assured us that they would not receive the antibiotics which they were routinely administered before slaughter, explaining that these were given so that the animals would not become ill before slaughter and would look their best! We could not believe what we had just heard and decided to research further.

Apparently, modern farming methods not only allow farmers to use antibiotics to help their investment to live longer and fight off disease, but also to use growth hormones to increase their size faster, both resulting in an increased risk of heart disease and cancer in humans who consume them. Additionally, doctors are over-prescribing antibiotics, so also adding antibiotics into the food chain must be detrimental to health.

Digestion of red meat is another problem. Digestion is a topic of its own and there is much to read and understand on how the human digestive system works and affects everything in the body. There is a modern day tendency to rush the eating of food and not chew it properly, so when this food is also difficult to digest the problem is exacerbated. Undigested food can lead to blockages in the colon — rotting, putrefying, fermenting and rancid food — and these blockages can sometimes sit in the colon for weeks, months and even longer. Some of this toxic debris can be forced through the walls of the colon along with the water and electrolytes, back into the blood stream, where it is seen by the immune system as a foreign invader. The immune system therefore attacks it and allergies are created, allergies which can result in a long list of other associated diseases culminating in serious and even life–threatening illness.

Another potential health risk is that when red meat is cooked at high temperatures it can result in a chemical change within the meat which causes the formation of carcinogens. Research suggests that by choosing lean cuts with the fat trimmed off and by grilling at a moderate heat, the risks of the carcinogens forming are reduced. Barbequing, deep frying and pan frying are the cooking methods most likely to produce carcinogens. There is evidence to suggest that the risk is reduced by marinating the meat first before cooking. Although much emphasis has been placed on the risks of eating red meat, the same risk of producing carcinogens when cooked at high temperatures was found in rotisserie chicken.

Joe ate much red meat before his diagnosis — he always pan

fried his meat and loved anything deep fried including fish and chips — but, after his diagnosis, when he ate meat as a treat (which was not often), he would pan fry it in coconut oil but he would never barbeque; in fact we stopped eating barbequed food altogether.

Sodas/Soft Drinks (diet/normal)

I recall on many supermarket trips filling the trolley a quarter full with fizzy drinks. Joe would drink at least three bottles a week and sometimes a bottle a day. Following our research he stopped them completely.

The sugar in soft drinks causes insulin to be released in the body to counteract the glucose in the drink and, whilst not causing cancer, sugar is its preferred energy source. In a recent study it was seen that men who drank just one fizzy drink a day were more likely to develop prostate cancer than those who refrained. Also, soft drinks have been linked to an increase in the risk of pancreatic cancer, the pancreas being the organ which produces insulin. Although fruit juices contain natural sugar these have not been linked to any increased risk.

White Foods

We avoided all white foods — white bread, white sugar, white pasta. They all lack basic nutrients needed for a healthy body and an efficient immune system. Eating too many white foods can suppress the immune system as the body is using valuable energy to process foods with little nutritional value when it needs this energy to process nutritional foods which will fuel the body and, over a period of time, this can leave the body vulnerable to attack.

Vegetable Oils

Vegetables oils are produced by extraction from seeds and margarine is made from these oils. They were practically non–existent in our diets until the early 1900's as the processes which are necessary to extract the oils were unknown before this time. The vegetable oils cannot be extracted naturally and so must be removed chemically, then deodorised and altered, creating some of the most chemically altered foods in most people's diets, yet they are promoted as healthy. Initially, we were also misled and were eating soya spread, until I learnt more about the facts surrounding margarine and spreads.

The majority of vegetable oils (at least in the US) are made from genetically engineered crops. They are also treated with herbicides and pesticides. As the oil is heated during cooking and mixes with oxygen, it becomes rancid. Eating foods cooked in these oils can seriously increase your risk of many degenerative diseases as oxidized cholesterol is introduced into the body.

It is essential for the human body to maintain a delicate balance of omega–3 and omega–6 fats as the body uses these to rebuild cells and for the production of hormones. Consequently, just like baking a cake, if the ingredients which are added together are incorrect in ratio, then the result will be wrong and inefficient. Therefore, introducing vegetable oils high in omega–6 fats into the body can throw this balance out. Omega–3 fats have been shown to help prevent cancer whereas omega–6 fats have been shown to increase the risk of cancer developing.

Vegetable oils are found in practically every processed food, and these oils are some of the most harmful substances which can be put into the body. It may be a simple decision to change the oil with which you cook to coconut oil and thereby avoid all of the aforementioned negatives of vegetable oils, but how do we avoid the foods manufactured using vegetable oils? Careful review of all food labels is a must and any foods which have soybean oil, vegetable oil or corn oil should be avoided. The main culprits are obvious — salad dressings, sauces, mayonnaise — but there are some surprises such as crisps, nuts, seeds, biscuits and crackers.

We cooked with olive oil for quite some time until we learnt that cooking with olive oil was not safe either, since once it is heated to high temperatures, olive oil can also become carcinogenic and lose all of its health benefits. Eventually we switched to organic coconut oil which is believed to be the safest oil with which to cook, in addition to being delicious and easily obtainable.

Margarine or Butter?

Vegetable oils are not naturally solid at cold temperatures and must be hydrogenated to accomplish this. During this process, those lovely unsaturated fats which we've heard so much about are created when the oils are subjected to extremely high temperatures. Additives and colours are added to improve the smell and appearance of the product.

We eventually switched to organic butter. Butter is a natural food and has many health benefits, but we always chose organic. Butter contains conjugated linoleic acid, which is a potent anti-cancer agent, muscle builder, and immunity booster. There are many further benefits to consuming butter but, as with all foods, it depends on your health issues as to whether this is good for your body e.g. butter is known to raise 'bad' cholesterol due to its saturated fat content.

Farmed Fish

Farmed fish are bred in a controlled environment, usually on the sea coast. They are bred in crowded conditions and, because of this, they are routinely given antibiotics in their food to prevent them from contracting diseases. They are fed on food which is sometimes made up of ground fish remains and PCBs (toxic pollutant known to cause cancer) as well as the antibiotics. Eating such toxins can obviously cause an increase of toxins in the body and hence increase the risk of cancer.

Crisps

The chemical acrylamide is found in crisps. This is known to cause nerve damage, and an excess of this in the body can contribute to cancer. Studies suggest that acrylamide is produced when foods high in carbohydrate are fried or baked. This chemical occurs in many foodstuffs, not just fried foods, but the levels are higher in fried foods. Although it is unlikely that the minimal levels of acrylamide found in the average person's diet would cause any problem whatsoever, because the immune system recognises this toxin and has to deal with it, it is still adding yet another burden to the immune system of a cancer patient.

Ice Cream

Ice-cream is mainly made from cow's milk. Most ice-cream contains carrageenan which is used mainly in dairy and meat products for its gelling and thickening properties. However, it can be found in a wide range of other foods. Research has suggested a link between this product and gastrointestinal cancers.

Canned and Processed Foods

We discarded all cans, even baked beans in cans. BPA, or Bisphenol A, is a toxic chemical that is used in most linings of food and drink cans and plastic bottles which can leak into the food or drink. BPA interferes with the endocrine system by mimicking the body's hormones, namely oestrogen. The endocrine system is a collection of glands that produce hormones which travel through the bloodstream and regulate your body's growth, metabolism and sexual functions. There is much research linking BPA with an increased risk of breast cancer and other illnesses.

There have been efforts to implement banning BPAs in America for several years and indeed Japan stopped using them in the '90s. Since breast cancer and prostate cancer are very much affected by hormones, it is especially relevant to patients with these cancers.

Ready Meals

We completely removed ready meals from our diet and cooked only fresh vegetables and fish, sometimes meat. Not only may there be harmful chemicals in the packaging, especially when heating in containers, but label reading can be horrifying. They are generally high in fat which can lead to obesity which is linked to an increased risk of cancer. Fat also alters the body's normal hormonal and chemical balances, sending signals which, under the right conditions, promote cancer growth.

Alcohol

Although this is categorised as an item which we avoided, in the beginning this was one of the things which Joe found most difficult to give up. Joe and I enjoyed a drink — we drank regularly and Joe sometimes drank *a lot!* However, towards the end of Joe's life, perhaps for the last year, he had no desire to drink alcohol and had by then drastically reduced his intake, drinking only whisky and Rioja red wine with an occasional beer as a treat.

Habitual drinking increases the risk of cancer, scientists believing that the increased risk comes when the body converts alcohol into acetaldehyde, a potent carcinogen, causing the liver to work hard to clear this toxin from the body. Cancers linked to alcohol use include the mouth, throat, voice box, oesophagus, liver, breast and colorectal region. Excess alcohol is unhealthy as it also weakens the immune system, which is the most important factor for good health and overcoming diseases, especially cancer. As a moderate drinker I can invariably feel the effects of alcohol on my immune system. Refraining from alcohol leads me to feel much more alive, focused and healthy, have more energy and better quality sleep.

Nuts

Peanuts contain many different mycotoxin–producing fungi and when we discovered this we stopped eating them. Ground or broken nuts (of any kind) are ready targets for airborne mould spores and quickly become rancid. Cashew nuts and dried coconut can similarly become contaminated and we avoided both of these also.

Sugary Breakfast Cereals

Joe loved cereals and it was difficult for him to cease eating them, but with great will he managed to eradicate them from his diet. Initially, we could not understand how cereals could be damaging — media actively encourages their consumption. For decades, we have been led to believe that a bowl of cereal is the best start to the day for your body, but for many cereals this is far from the truth.

Most cereals have large amounts of sugar pumped into them, sometimes as much as five teaspoons in a 40g serving when served with milk, and they have a very low nutritional value. Even muesli–type cereals can have a high sugar content. Also, unless the ingredients are organic, they will be subject to pesticide contamination. There has been much research linking sugary breakfast cereals and cancer, including one which demonstrates that a cardboard box can be more nutritious than a sugary breakfast cereal.

Cereal production generally requires high temperatures and during this process acrylamide is formed, one of the most potent cancer–causing agents. It is especially high in bran cereals as the temperature used to make these is higher than many others.

When I first learned how bad certain cereals are for your health, I threw out every box. Eggs, fruit, yoghurt or soaked and cooked porridge are much healthier breakfast options. Of course, there may be cereals on the market which are not produced by high temperature manufacturing processes which would not fall prey to these issues. My advice would be to actively seek confirmation of how the cereal was produced before purchasing.

Milk

We stopped drinking cow's milk and eating cow's cheese. Cows are injected with a genetically–engineered hormone which causes them to produce increased volumes of milk, but which also causes a rise in the growth hormone IGF–1 (insulin–growth factor 1). IGF–1 promotes cell division and prevents programmed cell death (apoptosis) which is the body's way of protecting against cancer. Cancer is encouraged by increased cell division and not allowing old cells to die. Pasteurisation does not kill IGF–1, nor does digestion. In addition, dairy cows are hooked by their udders to electronic milking machines that can cause the cow to suffer electric shocks, painful lesions and **mastitis**. Mastitis causes pus to be excreted by the udders which ends up in the milk and then in your body. To treat mastitis cows are injected with antibiotics.

Cows are milked for most days of the year, including when they are pregnant. Milk from a pregnant cow is especially bad for humans as it has increased levels of oestrogen and research shows that increased levels of oestrogen can increase the growth of certain cancers.

There are many alternatives available to cow's milk and, although it may take time to become accustomed to the taste, the health benefits are worth it. We mostly replaced cow's milk with soya milk. Like Marmite, most of the available alternatives you will either love or hate:

Soya	Creamy with a slightly nutty taste
Goat	Strong milk taste
Rice	Quite sweet tasting
Almond	Sweet almond tasting — can curdle in hot drinks
Hazelnut	Sweet and hazelnut tasting
Coconut	Quite similar in taste to skimmed milk and with only a light coconut flavour
Oat	Slightly sweet and neutral, but with a slight hint of oat

Additives

In addition to reviewing food labels for their nutritional content, we also reviewed them for additives and colours. It may be advisable to have extra garbage sacks to hand to use after reading this next article!

Below is an article which I found on the internet *(www. foodmatters.tv).* It is an extremely informative website packed with various printed and visual material of interest, and well worth a visit. This article details the top ten additives to avoid:

Unbelievably there are over three hundred chemicals used in processed foods today. These man–made chemicals are seen as foreign to our bodies, which often results in a number of implications to our health and well–being. Allergies are a common side–effect and monosodium glutamate, widely used in processed foods, is known to cause overeating and weight gain.

The best way to avoid exposure to these harmful chemicals is to understand the most common and dangerous additives and in which foods they are most often found. Here is our 'Top Ten Food Additives to Avoid' shopping guide.

- Artificial Sweeteners
- High Fructose Corn Syrup
- Monosodium Glutamate (MSG/E621)
- Trans Fat
- Common Food Dyes
- Sodium Sulphite (E221)
- Sodium Nitrate/Sodium Nitrite
- BHA and BHT (E320)
- Sulphur Dioxide (E220)
- Potassium Bromate

This is reproduced in full in Appendix 7.

By Laurentine ten Bosch and included by kind permission from Foodmatters.tv

Additives in Supplements

I always examine the contents of all vitamins and minerals for possible worrying additives such as bulkers and fillers. The manufacturers of supplements often add various fillers to their vitamin and mineral supplements to make production easier and faster and to make the tablets easier to swallow. This is no different to additives in food and they can be as harmful to your health. Although certain additives which we avoided may not be directly related to cancer, they can impede the response of the patient to treatments. It is extremely important to ensure that vitamins and supplements are only obtained from a supplier of high quality products as poor quality supplements add little or no nutritional value and may even be harmful. Additives which I looked out for and avoided were:

Hydrogenated Soybean Oil

In addition to the negative effects of hydrogenated oils already discussed, this oil is also widely used as a filler in vitamins and is obviously counter-productive to a supplement intended to improve health.

Magnesium Stearate

In research studies magnesium stearate has been linked to certain cancers. It is used as a lubricant during manufacture so that the vitamins do not stick to one another during production and the dose consistency is preserved. There has been research which has shown that it may cause a biofilm in the body which blocks it from absorbing needed nutrients. It has also been linked to suppression of the immune system.

Titanium Dioxide

This is an odourless, naturally-occurring mineral and is used in vitamins and cosmetics as a pigment. However, exposure to this metal can lead to problems with the immune system functionality. The International Agency for Research on Cancer *(www.iarc.fr)* has classified this substance as 'possibly carcinogenic to humans'. Obviously this decision would not have been taken lightly or without the existence of much research to support such a move. Its use is also regulated by the Food and Drugs Administration (FDA).

Silicon Dioxide

Silicon is essential to humans as it contributes to the health of bones and arteries. This is *not* to be confused with silicon dioxide. Silicon dioxide as a solid is found in nature as sand or quartz. However, amorphous silicon dioxide is used as a pesticide to kill insects, mites and ticks by removing their protective covering and causing them to dry out and die. Silicon dioxide is toxic, but because the amount which will be ingested due to pesticides used on foodstuffs is so negligible to humans, there have been no restrictions put upon its use. Crystalline silicon dioxide is known to cause silicosis which may lead to lung cancer, but there has been no such link with amorphous silicon dioxide. It is used as an anti-caking product in the production of vitamins and supplements to stop them from sticking together.

Sodium Aluminium

Used to speed up the production of a vitamin tablet, sodium aluminium is basically aluminium and therefore a neurotoxin and a known cause of Alzheimer's disease.

Sodium Benzoate

This is a further additive which we avoided. It is used as a preservative in the production of liquid vitamins and is most frequently found in mineral and juice drinks. When it comes into contact with an acid e.g. citric acid or ascorbic acid (vitamin C) it forms benzene which is a known carcinogen. The instructions on its storage advise that it should not be kept near foods and beverages, so how can it be safe as an additive?

Talc

Talc is a known carcinogen and is also used as a filler (binds the supplement together) in the manufacture of supplements.

Cookwear

We threw out all of our non-stick pans as, when heated to very high temperatures, certain non-stick coatings can emit extremely toxic fumes which can be re-ingested.

We also threw out all of our aluminium pans as aluminium

can be dissolved into foods when cooking, especially when cooking acidic foods. We only cooked with stainless steel pans.

The Microwave

Before Joe was diagnosed with cancer we, like millions of other households, owned and used a microwave, although I never liked the idea of microwaved foods and never ate anything from the microwave myself. I do, however, remember preparing chips in a box for the children in the microwave. During my research following the diagnosis, I found some disturbing facts about microwaves.

After conducting their own research, the Russians banned microwave ovens in 1976, later lifting the ban during Perestroika. They issued an international warning about possible biological and environmental damage associated with the use of microwave ovens. Russian investigators had found that carcinogens were formed from the microwaving of nearly all foods tested. The microwaving of milk and grains converted some of the amino acids into carcinogenic substances. Microwaving prepared meats caused the formation of the cancer–causing agents D–nitrosodienthanolamines. Thawing frozen fruit by microwave converted their glucoside and galactoside fractions into carcinogenic substances. Extremely short exposure to the microwave of raw, cooked or frozen vegetables converted their plant alkaloids into carcinogens.

A Swiss scientist studied the effects of microwaved foods and found that microwave cooking changes the nutrients in food. It also causes changes in the blood when these foods are eaten which have negative effects on health. Even standing in front of a microwave is damaging to your health as microwaves can leak from the oven into your body.

Another problem with microwave ovens is that carcinogenic toxins can leak out of the plastic or paper containers or covers into the food.

Sodium Lauryl Sulphate

This chemical is found in a wide variety of shampoos and soaps. Its main use is as a very strong degreaser and floor cleaner which is an irritant. It is used in shampoos and soaps simply because it is cheap, but the process which is used to make the chemical useful in production can create 1,4–dioxane which *is* harmful and also a hormone disrupter; a problem with hormone-linked cancers. Agencies around the world have stated that there is no link between sodium lauryl sulphate and cancer. Whilst it is accepted that in itself it is not carcinogenic, it is nonetheless a chemical which is being applied to the body which the immune system must fend off and should, therefore, be avoided.

Parabens

These are chemicals used as preservatives by cosmetic and pharmaceutical industries. Ethyl–, butyl–, methyl– and propyl–parabens are examples of parabens commonly used in cosmetics and personal care products. Used to prevent the growth of microbes in products and extend shelf life, they can be absorbed through the skin and have been found in biopsies from breast tissue tumours. They have been linked to cancer, skin irritation, immunotoxicity and neurotoxity and are also known to disrupt hormone function. I avoid all parabens and only buy organic, paraben–free products.

Useful Resources

There are so many changes which can be made to a lifestyle in order to improve health and well–being and assessing which changes are needed requires guidance. I found the Life Extension site *(www.lef.org)* an amazing resource for information relating to new discoveries in health, nutrition and anti–ageing supplements. Subscription is very reasonable. It is less than one hundred pounds to become a member and you receive a monthly magazine with all of the latest medical and anti–ageing news. It proved to be invaluable. They are US–based but deliver speedily to England, also delivering high quality supplements at very reasonable prices, especially for members. Also available is access to a phone line where members can speak with health advisors and medical doctors about their nutrition and health concerns but since I did not use this service I cannot comment on its usefulness. The Life Extension Foundation is the world's largest organisation dedicated to finding scientific methods for addressing disease, ageing and death. It is a non–profit making organisation which funds pioneering scientific research aimed at achieving an indefinitely extended healthy human lifespan. The fruits of this research are used to develop novel disease prevention and treatment protocols.

Included with kind permission from Life Extension

I also subscribe to the Prostate Cancer Research Institute (*www.prostate-cancer.org*). It is free to subscribe and I receive a monthly magazine with all of the latest developments and findings on prostate cancer which I also found very useful. It is called 'PCRI Insights Magazine'. It is delivered by email or, upon request, can be delivered by post.

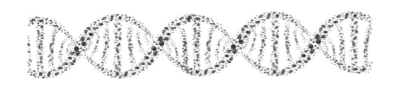

11 — Supplements, Cleanses and Treatments

There are many supplements and cleanses which we tried. Not all of them will be suitable for all people — it was very much a case of trial and error. The following were treatments which we felt were effective for Joe.

There are sufficient testimonies and positive research results which make it worth having confidence in researching, and perhaps trying, alternative diets or treatments, but only ever after agreement from your medical professional — this is imperative as differing treatments can have negative effects when combined, and can be contraindicative (act against each other) — so always seek advice first.

Doctor Young

www.phmiracleliving.com

Greens Drink

I would insist that Joe drank his greens drink daily, which he hated, but he co-operated as he knew that it was good for him and continued to take this long-term. When Joe was sticking to the greens drinks and the diet, it felt like his condition was under control. I believe that this was a crucial factor in Joe's prolonged good health. The greens drink was an inexpensive but effective way to improve Joe's energy levels. Towards the end I also began to add Turmeric drops to the drink for extra impact.

The greens drink alkalises the body, gives nutrition and creates energy and health. It is green–chlorophyll rich which builds blood and keeps it healthy. The greens drinks were made using Dr Young's products. There are other products on the market which are similar, but in my opinion Dr Young is an expert in this field. Dr Young has also written a number of books on the subject of PH balance, diet and health, his most well-known to date probably being 'The PH Miracle'. In my opinion, this is a must read for every cancer patient. Non-cancer readers who decide to follow his advice may be surprised when they unexpectedly regain lost vigour and body shape.

So how is the greens drink prepared? I used:

2 scoops of doc broc power plants
1 scoop of phour salts
5 PH drops
1 scoop of soya sprouts
1 scoop of TerraPHirma clay

Add together in a safe (no BPA in the lining) plastic bottle, shake well and it is ready to drink. It is best prepared immediately prior to drinking and should be drunk as rapidly as is possible without causing discomfort. Occasionally, during the latter days when effort was tiring, Joe found it difficult to drink this so I would give him a spoonful of bicarbonate of soda as an alternative.

Doc Broc Power Plants

A mixture of vibrant and energising green power plants, organic vegetables, fruits and grasses such as kale, okra, avocado, cucumber and wheatgrass. It is prepared at low temperatures so that the essential nutrients in the food are preserved. When you take a scoop of doc broc power plants you can see the particles jumping off the scoop like electricity before your eyes. They contain much chlorophyll, which builds up the blood, and are very alkalising.

Young Phorever Phour Salts

Young pHorever pHour Salts is a combination of four powerful carbonate salts (sodium bicarbonate, magnesium bicarbonate, potassium bicarbonate and calcium bicarbonate) which help to maintain the alkaline design of human, plant and animal organisms. These salts are naturally occurring in all fluids of the body. Specifically, they can aid in the reduction of acidity in the lymphatic, circulatory and gastrointestinal systems. Consequently, this reduces acidity in the body, organs and cells.

Terra pHirma Clay

Terra pHirma clay is Montmorillonite Clay, named after the location of the deposit where it was first identified — near Montmorillon, France. This clay provides an impressive assortment of alkalising minerals, including calcium, iron, magnesium, potassium, manganese, sodium, sulphur and silica. Furthermore, these minerals in clay exist in natural proportion to one another, so they are more easily and thoroughly absorbed by the body. The minerals in this clay are also highly negatively charged — full of electrons that absorb, adsorb (to hold molecules of a gas or liquid as a thin film on the outside surface or internal surfaces of a material) and eliminate many positively–charged toxins in the body. In fact, this clay can absorb and adsorb many times its weight in acids, holding them until your body can safely eliminate them. Terra pHirma is truly the earth's natural acid absorber and adsorber and can be used to neutralise over–acidity internally (digestive tract) as well as externally (skin). Montmorillonite Clay provides a range of benefits including improved digestion and elimination, better circulation, higher quality sleep, increased energy, decreased emotional abnormality, stronger immune system, weight loss, balanced sugar level and more.

PuripHy PH Drops

PuripHy is water purification in a bottle. With just a few drops, PuripHy acts as an antioxidant, neutralising algaes, bacteria, yeasts, moulds, parasites and mycotoxins. Furthermore, PuripHy is an oxygen catalyst, helping your blood absorb more oxygen from the water you drink. This is achieved as PuripHy optimizes the water by decreasing hydrogen ions and increasing hydroxyl ions.

PuripHy is a combination of liquid sodium bicarbonate, potassium bicarbonate and potassium hydroxide. PuripHy can be added to liquids to help to reduce dietary acids in the stomach and small and large intestine and to rid the water of harmful bacteria, yeast and mould. PuripHy also helps to buffer the stomach acids of hydrochloric acid which can lead to acid reflux and heartburn. It helps to protect the alkaline environment of the alimentary canal from dietary acids, especially the small intestine and the delicate intestinal villi.

Biolive Soya Sprouts

These are a good source of organic plant protein, which increases energy and contains unique protective compounds to detoxify the blood. They are also packed with soya isoflavones, a known antioxidant, which protects the cells from damage.

Included with kind permission from Doctor Young

AlgaeCal

www.algaecal.com

Algae Cal Plus

Calcium was obviously a high priority for Joe since the cancer had already spread to his bones when he was diagnosed. Calcium is essential for strong teeth and bones and is obtained by dietary methods by consuming milk, yoghurt, cheese, dark green vegetables, peas, beans and nuts.

I would give Algae Cal to Joe when I was not giving him Theta liquid minerals. Most calcium supplements are produced from ground rock or chalk and usually have additives pumped into them. Algae Cal is completely different. This wild–harvested, plant–sourced calcium is derived from South American marine algae called Algas Calcareas. The entire kiwi–fruit size algae ball is hand–harvested, sun–dried, then milled into a powder. There is no extraction process used, nor additives — just pure whole food. The Algae Cal marine plant draws calcium and seventy other minerals from sea water and pre–digests it for you, much like a carrot or potato root breaks down the inedible rock minerals in soil, converting them into a useable form which your body recognises as food. Algae Cal plant–digested calcium is so body–friendly that 97% of Algae Cal's calcium goes into solution in thirty minutes using U.S. Pharmacopeial Convention (USP) standard tests simulating stomach conditions — proving that it is very bio–accessible.

Included with kind permission from AlgaeCal

Empirical Labs

www.empirical-labs.com

Omnizyme

Omnizyme is a digestive enzyme which Joe would take an hour before heavier meals. This is a well–balanced, plant–based, digestive enzyme formula. Prior to writing this book, I didn't realise how many key roles digestive enzymes fulfill in the body, or that the body's natural ability to make digestive enzymes decreases with each year that passes. Enzymes are produced in the pancreas and other endocrine glands, and are produced in raw foods which we eat. Unfortunately, in today's environment, diets consist of processed foods, overcooked foods and not enough raw foods. In addition, lifestyles are so busy that food is not chewed for long enough causing a lack of essential digestive enzymes and undigested foods. Digestive enzymes help to reduce joint and muscle inflammation and act as a natural pain reliever. They also help to remove toxins and other debris in the circulatory system and can help to stimulate immune response. Hence they are very important for cancer patients with weakened immune systems and often impaired digestion.

Liposomal Vitamin C

Empirical Labs has mastered liposomal technology using natural phosphatidylcholine liposomes as a delivery method for vitamin C. They believe that each and every component of their products must be as health building as possible. Current literature has shown that hydrogenated liposomes strongly increase LDL (bad) cholesterol levels while natural non–hydrogenated phosphatidylcholine was shown not to alter cholesterol levels in primates. Empirical Labs are currently the only company to use all natural non–hydrogenated phosphatidylcholine as a delivery system. The product has only what is needed:

- Vitamin C (as sodium ascorbate) which is nutrition
- Natural phosphatidylcholine (delivery method and nutrition)
- Purified water
- Natural flavours and a preservative

Empirical Labs take great care to process their liposomes properly in order to generate correctly structured spherical liposomes in their product. If the structure is not there, they are not liposomes.

Included with kind permission from Empirical Labs

Dulwich Health

www.dulwichhealth.com

Seagreens

This unique, wild wrack seaweed grows in the crystal clear Arctic water among remote conservation islands over sixty miles from the coast of Norway. It is hand–harvested, air–dried and immediately milled. Seagreens is pure seaweed and contains three different varieties of wrack not found in any other seaweed product. Seagreens contains all of the micro–nutrients missing from processed foods and depleted soil. It contains over one hundred vitamins, minerals, trace elements, amino acids and valuable compounds. It also contains just enough iodine to regulate the thyroid and metabolism on a continuous basis. It is used to strengthen immunity, improve resistance to disease and aid recovery.

Included with kind permission from Dulwich Health

Allera Health

www.allerahealth.com

Immune Extra

ImmuneExtra is an all–natural, vegetarian, clinically–tested supplement containing Proligna, an all–natural, preservative–free, patented, botanical compound, first studied in Japan and developed by scientists at the Tampa Bay Research Institute in Florida.

ImmuneExtra uses pine cone extract which has been used in Japan for centuries for the treatment of a myriad of ailments. It is used to enhance and support the immune system which is a vitally important concern for anyone fighting any disease. It can also be taken as a preventative measure to help to ensure that the immune system is strong enough to keep disease at bay.

Included with kind permission from Allera Health

Allicin International Limited

www.allicin.co.uk

Allicin

In common with other plants, garlic has its own defence mechanism and, when it is injured, garlic produces allicin which is, in effect, a natural insecticide. Unfortunately, no clinical trials have taken place on it as it is so unstable that it is difficult to obtain accurate data.

Allicin International Limited has devised a manufacturing process where the allicin is stabilised and made available in various forms. It is especially effective when the immune system is depleted and provides an extremely effective boost. Also, when Joe had bacteria in his blood (which was visible under the microscope), I would give him Allicin and within a few weeks a new analysis would always show that the bacteria had cleared. I have given this supplement to relatives with illnesses for which they had been prescribed antibiotics and Allicin works when antibiotics are ineffective. I continue to take it on a regular basis to prevent illness.

Included with kind permission from Allicin International Ltd

The Wolfe Clinic

www.thewolfeclinic.com
www.shopthewolfeclinic.com

DMSO and Cesium Chloride

DMSO (Dimethyl sulfoxide) is a strong anti–inflammatory agent, a strong immune stimulant and an antioxidant, free radical scavenger. It is also a vasodilator (it opens up the small blood vessels in the body), commonly used to stimulate immunity in cancer patients and to assist with immune suppressive conditions, chronic fatigue syndrome and AIDS. It is a most useful anti–inflammatory treatment for arthritic patients, as well as being effective against degenerative diseases. DMSO is thought to be a safe and effective therapy.

Through my endless researching I came across the Wolfe Clinic which offered this protocol (treatment programme), consisting of cesium chloride, DMSO, a combination of theta minerals, vitamin supplements and amino acids. It seemed too good to be true, and although it sounded a little scary to administer, I was eager for Joe to try it. The reason for my trepidation was that I was advised to have Joe's blood analysed regularly whilst using it to monitor changes in the electrolytes, minerals and uric acid as these could become out of balance and the uric acid levels could become too high which would cause damage to the kidneys. Furthermore, dangerous changes in the potassium levels could lead to other health risks.

The idea behind this treatment is that DMSO is used as a vehicle to carry the cesium chloride to the cancer cells and this allows the cesium chloride to more easily penetrate the cancer cells in order to raise the alkalinity of the cell's PH. This sudden rise in alkalinity should destroy any cancer cells in a few days.

I first tried this protocol on Joe towards the end of July 2009 when he was taking the tablet form of chemotherapy, which was at that time not working and not slowing the cancer. Unfortunately, Joe could not tolerate the DMSO and Cesium at all at this time and it made him violently sick, so I decided to leave it and try it another time when he was undergoing no other treatments. I was extremely disappointed because, according to my research, it seemed like the miracle cure for which we had been waiting. I even tried to reduce the amount of cesium chloride and DMSO to see if Joe would be more tolerant to smaller doses, but this was also intolerable. It must have been the cesium which Joe could not tolerate as he had regularly been administered DMSO intravenously with his vitamin C, but then again the DMSO and cesium were now being administered into the stomach which could potentially have been the cause of the sickness. At a later time I tried this protocol again but the reaction was the same, which seemed strange as Joe could tolerate most things and responded well to most treatments with few side-effects, but not this one.

Theta Liquid Minerals

The human body is made up of many minerals which need to be kept at certain levels for the body to function efficiently. Because Theta minerals are in liquid form, they proved to be invaluable when Joe did not feel like taking any tablets but needed the mineral and trace element boost, especially when he was on chemotherapy.

The Wolfe Clinic's Theta Minerals dietary supplements are the purest minerals which I could find on the market (up to 99.9999% pure) in the purest water (a five step purification process assures absolutely pure water). Theta Minerals, through a complex proprietary process, liquefy minerals to a state where (when dehydrated) they will grow crystals. This process duplicates nature's method of turning minerals from the earth into a form useable by man, just like plants process minerals from the earth, the minerals being changed to the crystalline form necessary for absorption by the body.

Recognition of the importance of the minerals required for perfect health is so new that few textbooks contain much about it. It is now believed that at least twenty–four elements are essential to living matter i.e. deficiency symptoms occur when these elements are lacking and then resolve when proper balance is achieved. Minerals are essential to physical and mental health. They are a basic part of all cells, particularly blood, nerve, muscle, bones, teeth and soft tissue. Some are essential for functional support, such as the electrolyte minerals e.g. sodium, potassium, and chloride, which help to regulate the fluid and acid–base balance of our bodies. Other minerals are part of enzymes that catalyze biochemical reactions, aid energy production, metabolism, nerve transmission, muscle contraction and cell permeability. Carbohydrates, proteins, fats, vitamins and minerals are the building blocks of our diet and provide the fuel, or source of energy, to maintain life and promote cell and tissue growth and other biochemical support.

Minerals contain no calories or energy in them, coming from the earth and eventually return to the earth, but they assist the body in energy production. They can most simply be defined as chemical molecules that cannot be reduced to simpler substances. They exist in their inorganic state in the earth, and in their organic state as the basic constituent of all living matter. The main elements essential to health, each of which makes up more than .01% of total body weight, are termed macro–minerals (calcium, phosphorus, chlorine, potassium, sulphur, sodium, magnesium and silicon). The next group of elements, termed micro–minerals or trace minerals, each constitute less than .01% of total body weight, but they are also essential to health. These are iron, copper, zinc, iodine, cobalt, bromide, boron, manganese, selenium, fluorine, molybdenum, vanadium, arsenic and chromium. Other elements contained in the body include some of the toxic metals (lead, aluminium, cadmium, and mercury).

Theta Potassium

Potassium is called the alkalizer as it neutralises acids and restores alkaline salts to the blood stream. It works with sodium in all cells, including nerve synapses, to maintain and restore membrane potentials and assist in metabolic processes. Potassium is critical to cardiovascular and nerve function, regulating the transfer of nutrients into cells, and for muscle energy. Potassium also regulates water balance, assists recuperative powers, aids rheumatic or arthritic conditions (causes acids to leave joints and ease stiffness), is vital for elimination of wastes, is a natural pain desensitizer, helps control convulsions, headaches and migraines, promotes faster healing of cuts, bruises & other injuries and generally contributes to a sense of well–being. Potassium is stored in the muscles.

Joe was quite often low on potassium due to episodes of diarrhoea and sickness and often needed to supplement his levels. The Theta liquid minerals were fantastic as, when Joe was not up to taking many tablets, I could combine all of the theta minerals together and he could drink this quite easily and it never bothered him.

Normally, a potassium intake sufficient to support everyday life for healthy human beings can be obtained from a good diet. Foods rich in potassium are potatoes, bananas, dried apricots, nuts, chocolate, avocados, soya beans and bran, although it is also present in fish, meat, fruit and vegetables in sufficient quantities.

Theta Magnesium

Magnesium is a natural tranquilizer. Called the 'anti–stress mineral', it aids in relaxing nerves, relieving tension, assisting digestion, activating enzymes important for protein and carbohydrate metabolism and modulating the electrical potential across all cell membranes. It is important in the production and transfer of energy, muscle contraction and relaxation, and nerve conduction. It also aids regularity, is necessary to keep vertebrae in their proper position, induces restful sleep, purifies and purges body tissues (combats acids, toxins, gases, impurities, and neutralizes poisons) and lowers fever. Magnesium is stored in the bowel, nerves and ligaments.

Hundreds of enzymes require magnesium enzymes to function. As with potassium, a normal healthy diet would never result in a magnesium deficiency. Nuts, coffee, cocoa, tea, oats, green leafy vegetables, fish and honey are all good sources for magnesium.

Side–effects from cancer treatments such as diarrhoea and sickness could reduce levels of magnesium, as could poor food intake, poor nutrition and a weakened immune system.

Theta Super Silver

There are three main grades of processed silver (cilver) — colloidal silver, ionic silver and super cilver.
See Appendix 8 for full description.

Theta Selenium

Selenium is an essential trace mineral that works with vitamin E in metabolic functions. It promotes normal body growth, fertility, encourages tissue elasticity and is a potent antioxidant that naturally reduces the retention of toxic metals in the body. Selenium is crucial for the proper functioning of the heart muscle and there is evidence that it can help the body to fight cancer with low soil levels of selenium having long been associated with higher cancer rates. Selenium is stored in muscle and other tissues, as well as in the liver and kidneys.

Theta Germanium

Germanium is one of the most dynamic new discoveries in the realm of trace elements necessary for optimum nutritional health. Germanium raises the level of activity of various organs (facilitates oxygen uptake) and helps to expel harmful pollutants and arrest germ activity. Germanium serves as an electrical semi–conductor; it helps correct distortions in the electrical fields of the body.

Germanium is still being researched for all of its possible supplementary applications. A poor immune system, low energy and cancer indicate germanium deficiencies. It is believed to act as an anti–cancer agent and is effective for viral, bacterial and fungal infections.

Niacin

Niacin is one of the B vitamins that has been shown to provide multiple health benefits and may be a helpful supplement in fighting cancer. Also known as vitamin B3, it helps the body to create energy from carbohydrates like any other B vitamin, helps improve circulation and lowers cholesterol levels.

This was added intravenously to Joe's Vitamin C and DMSO drip every two weeks.

Included with kind permission from the Wolfe Clinic

Various Sources Available

Vitamin D

The importance of vitamin D supplement becomes increasingly evident every day, not only for cancer sufferers but for everyone. It is the most talked about and written about supplement of the decade. Whilst studies continue to refine optimal blood levels and recommended dietary amounts, the fact remains that a huge part of the population are deficient in this essential nutrient. Vitamin D is important for overall health, making strong bones, helping the body to repair and fight off illnesses, maintaining a balance between calcium and phosphorus in the body and controlling how many of these nutrients are absorbed through foods.

Growing evidence confirms that good vitamin D status decreases the risk for many cancers. It can also improve the results of chemotherapy by making the cancer more sensitive to this treatment and it is known to slow the growth of the cancer, thereby extending the survival period in people who already have the disease. Recent and ongoing studies prove that vitamin D is a key player in cancer prevention, having been shown to contain anti–tumour and anti–inflammatory properties. It has also been shown to interfere with oestrogen synthesis, which impedes cancer's growth.

There are two main ways of providing the body with vitamin D. Known as 'the sunshine vitamin,' it is acquired naturally through the skin from the sun's rays. The less sun exposure and the more sunscreen used, the lower the levels of vitamin D. Exposure to the sun without sun protection would be one method, but definitely not a good idea since this is a known cause of skin cancer. The other method of obtaining vitamin D is by supplementing. Unfortunately, it is difficult to get enough vitamin D from our diet as there is only a small amount of vitamin D in a few foods, which include salmon, mackerel, tuna, sardines, beef liver, egg yolks and cod liver oil.

I believe that our trips contributed to Joe's extended life and he always felt much better when he had time in the sunshine. Towards the end of his life the long flights would bring on bouts of pain, but he was prepared to deal with the discomfort in exchange for some time soaking up the sun's warmth.

Royal Jelly

This was one supplement which Joe decided that he wanted to take. It was not often that Joe decided he wanted to take anything, but he liked the sound of a natural product that was likely to give him more energy which is precisely what royal jelly claims to do; give more energy, stamina and vitality. Joe said that he felt the benefit from taking this and had improved energy levels and stamina.

Royal jelly is extremely rich in nutrients with an average serving containing seventeen different amino acids and most of the B vitamins. It also contains iron and calcium, together with vitamins A, C and E, which have the ability to cancel out free radical activity which is obviously of benefit to cancer patients. It has anti–bacterial properties, improves the health of the blood and, most importantly for a cancer patient, it has been shown in tests to restrict the flow of blood to tumours.

Aspirin

Unfortunately, I did not come across aspirin in my research until after Joe had passed away. It would have been most effective and may have prevented the deep–vein thrombosis which Joe developed as it slows down the time that blood takes to thicken and clot. There has been much research and evidence to indicate that aspirin slows down the spread of cancer and may even help in its prevention.

When the body is functioning normally without injury, COX–1 (cyclooxygenase–1) produces prostaglandins, which are like hormones, as a normal function. They are quickly broken down by the body. However, when the body is injured the COX–2 enzyme releases extra prostaglandins which then cause inflammation and pain at the source of the injury as part of the body's natural healing process. If too many prostaglandins are released then unwanted inflammation and pain are created. The overproduction of these prostaglandins and over–inflammation can inadvertently set off steps towards cancer development such as cell division, prevention of apoptosis and metastasis. Aspirin is a COX–2 inhibitor and consequently helps to prevent the onset of this process by making it difficult for too many prostaglandins to be produced. It has been used in the control of colon and breast cancers.

Probiotic

Probiotics are organisms, often described as good or friendly bacteria, which are introduced into the body as supplements to help to protect us from unfriendly micro–organisms which can lead to disease.

Taking a good probiotic daily can help to improve the immune system and maintain intestinal balance by introducing good bacteria into the gut. Towards the end, Joe was constantly taking antibiotics, which can reduce the friendly bacteria in our bodies as they kill good and bad bacteria, and his immune system was also weakened as, when we have more bad bacteria than good, the immune system has to work extra hard to eliminate it. A lack of good bacteria can lead to digestive and urinary tract problems such as diarrhoea and yeast infections.

Joe always suffered from diarrhoea, even more so when having chemotherapy and probiotics improved his condition.

Wheatgrass

Wheatgrass contains multiple health benefits — it is a powerful, detoxifying food which strengthens the immune system, helps to purify the blood and protect it, helps to restore alkalinity to the blood and strengthen the cells. It is packed with vitamins, minerals and amino acids. There is a strong interest in the US where outlets have sprung up serving this as a drink along with other health drinks and foods.

We bought a wheatgrass sprouter in an attempt to grow our own wheatgrass. Unfortunately it proved difficult to grow and so we progressed to ordering in fresh wheatgrass already grown in trays — all that we had to do was cut it and squeeze it. However, we again found this to be a strain on our time and squeezing it was just not practical with our busy lives and travel schedules. So we found that the best solution was to order in organic freeze dried powder and we added one teaspoon to the daily greens drink. I discovered more recently that fresh frozen wheatgrass is readily available to buy on the internet in individual portion pots. I put one of these in a blender with fresh apple juice for a refreshing drink.

Sodium Bicarbonate

I gave Joe Sodium Bicarbonate orally, particularly when he had heartburn or acidic conditions. I would give him one heaped teaspoon in a glass of warm water daily, sometimes twice daily, sometimes for periods of a month. It kept Joe's body alkaline and never upset him. If I was on a low budget then I would definitely use this for a longer period as the cost is negligible.

I heard an account from an old gentleman who had two old dears as his neighbours. He wrote that they lived to be ninety six and one hundred years old having both taken one third teaspoon of sodium bicarbonate every night before retiring to bed in a glass of tepid water.

Sodium Bicarbonate has been used as an alternative treatment for many years and there is much research to suggest that it is particularly effective in the treatment of cancer. It is also found in the corridors of orthodox oncology where it is used to keep the toxic chemotherapy agents from killing people too quickly, saving countless lives every day. A deficiency of bicarbonate ions in the body contributes to a range of diseases and medical conditions.

Turmeric

Early stage research has taken place to carry out trials using turmeric, a spice used in making curry which contains the chemical curcumin, to help to combat bowel cancer. Bowel cancer is particularly difficult to treat as patients are unable to tolerate repeated rounds of chemotherapy due to the extreme side-effects, and quite often the chemotherapy is ineffective. Curcumin has been shown to make the cancer cells more sensitive to chemotherapy which in turn means that lower doses can be given to patients who can then have the chemotherapy for longer periods. In early stage results it has also been shown to slow down metastasis in prostate cancer patients. Curcumin has antioxidant and anti-inflammatory properties.

Detox

When we began our journey to better health, I searched for a way to eliminate bacterias, parasites, moulds and yeasts from the body so that the detoxification process would be quicker. Although it would be impossible to eliminate all parasites from the body, as it is quite normal to have a small number of them, it is important to eliminate as many as possible on a regular basis. We pick up these invaders every day by way of the things which we eat, drink and touch. These parasites use our nutrients to survive, and this can cause acidic conditions leading to sickness or disease as well as being an ever-present strain on the immune system.

The first type of detox which we followed was a programme to eliminate bacterias, parasites (such as the parasites which cause viruses), moulds and yeasts known as a parasite cleansing programme. Hulda Clark discovered this herbal parasite cleanse.

Hulda Clark is now deceased. However, her work continues and you can find Dr. Clark's information centre online at _www. drclark.net_.

The herbal parasite cleanse comprises of wormwood capsules, clove capsules and black walnut tincture. These three herbs are used together to ensure elimination of all stages of the unwanted parasites. Full details of the programme can be found at _www.drclark.net/ cleanses_, or by reading 'The Cure For All Cancers' by Hulda Clark. This was a treatment which we performed every six months to begin with and then at least once a year.

As part of the programme we would always perform a liver cleanse after the herbal parasite cleanse. This comprised of fresh grapefruit juice, Epsom salts and olive oil (thin, good-tasting olive oil is best). It is quite revolting and if you do not stick to the programme exactly then you can feel quite unwell — indeed not everyone can manage the liver cleanse but Joe and I did not have a problem with it. According to Dr Clark, 'cleaning the liver bile ducts is the most powerful procedure that you can do to improve your body's health. But it should not be done before the parasite programme'. After carrying out the herbal parasite cleanse and liver cleanse programme we would follow up with the weekly maintenance parasite cleanse programme, which is explained on Hulda Clark's website, for another month. We would be quite tired whilst undertaking this treatment — I would do the programme with Joe to encourage him, but also to obtain the benefits for myself. The very first time that we followed the treatment my daughter and son also joined in. We all felt the effects and were quite tired, but once the process was complete we felt recharged and energised.

According to Dr Clark 'for many persons, including children, the biliary tubing is choked with gallstones. Some develop allergies or hives but some have no symptoms. When the gallbladder is scanned or X-rayed nothing is seen. Typically they are not in the gallbladder. Not only that, most are too small and not calcified, a pre-requisite for visibility on X-ray. There are over half a dozen varieties of gallstones, most of which have cholesterol crystals in them. They can be black, red, white, green or tan coloured. The black stones are full of lubricating fluid. The green ones get their colour from being coated in bile. As the stones grow and become more numerous, the back pressure on the liver causes it to make less bile. It is also thought to slow the flow of lymphatic fluid'.

We were first advised to follow the liver cleanse treatment by Dr Hilu. During a routine check of Joe's blood, Dr Hilu observed an enormous parasite which we presumed had been caused by raw seafood which Joe had eaten. We therefore did as we were told and performed the parasite cleanse followed by the liver cleanse. He told us that we would be amazed by how many stones would come out of our bodies. Gosh he was right! The following day Joe passed hundreds of green stones, too many to count. I also passed well over a hundred stones along with hundreds of minute small white balls, chaff or cholesterol crystals. But, after many years of performing these treatments, I am lucky to get any stones out at all.

We always followed the liver cleanse with a course of Oxytech which is a product available from Dulwich Health (_www. dulwichhealth.co.uk_). It helps to eliminate candida, bloated stomach, irritable bowel, leaky gut, skin disorders, continuous constipation or diarrhoea and lack of oxygen and energy. It is like a colonic without the pipe and much gentler, breaking down debris in the colon into very small pieces so that it can be more easily eliminated. After two weeks of taking this product we would be feeling great. We also did this every six months.

Detoxing and cleansing were effective whilst Joe's body was strong enough to cope with the treatments, but we did not carry out any of them whilst Joe was undergoing intravenous chemotherapy, except for the greens drinks and supplements.

Included by kind permission from Dr. Clark Information Centre

Geopathic Stress

It has been confirmed by many doctors and therapists that Geopathic Stress must be cleared before any cancer treatment can be one hundred percent successful. Many eminent doctors who specialise in cancer have associated cancer directly with Geopathic Stress, so this is not simply some hocus–pocus treatment.

Joe's sleeping patterns were always bad and he often woke several times throughout the night, finding it difficult to go back to sleep as thoughts of work would immediately invade his consciousness. Often he would sit up and watch television — we had a huge television in the bedroom as well as CCTV monitors which were left on all night and I could never sleep well, always feeling tired even if I had managed to have a relatively good night's sleep. So I began to research possible causes of bad sleeping patterns.

Geopathic Stress ('geo' from the Greek word for earth and 'pathic' from the Greek word pathos meaning to suffer, cause disease) is the study of how the earth and its energy can affect human health. The earth's vibrations are constant and continually rise up through the earth. However, when these vibrations become disturbed and distorted, they can affect the human body in a negative way. It is by no means a new concept and these vibrations have always been part of our lives.

In ancient China, Feng Shui was very much a part of everyday life, and now, after almost three thousand years, this science is experiencing a rebirth, as is the science of Geopathic Stress.

The earth has strong magnetic currents running throughout, and it is well–known that water interferes with this energy field. If a person passes over an area where underground water is interfering with the earth's natural vibrations then there would be little or no consequence. However, if a person is sleeping above such interference then this can affect a human by lowering the effectiveness of the immune system. Everybody is different and will react in a different way to the disturbance, some not at all. In today's modern world it may be difficult to accept this as a concept, but daily it becomes more acceptable and anything which *can* help to improve physical well–being is worth investigating and laying skepticism aside.

Basically, various underground formations, such as subterranean water currents, specific mineral deposits, or different fault lines emit specific electromagnetic fields that can be harmful for a human dwelling as they interfere with the natural vibrations of the earth, and the people living therein can be affected by the disturbance but not feel it. In the case of underground running water, an electromagnetic field is created in the opposite direction to its flow by friction, which then creates strong, unhealthy energy flows. Surface water does not normally create stress.

I decided that there was sufficient documentary evidence to investigate further and so I called an expert dowser from the south of England, Sussex, a man called Roy Riggs (www.royriggs.co.uk). He arrived by train and I collected him from the station. He came equipped with his dowsing equipment which looked like a pair of knitting needles and a pendulum. He tested every room inside the house and then he tested my son's house, my daughter's house (which are both on our land) and outside my house. He concluded that our bed was sitting directly above an underwater stream and advised that we should move immediately out of that bedroom and into another bedroom in the house. When we bought the house we were made aware that we were sitting on an underground well, but we did not know about the underwater stream running under our house and the damage that it could cause. It ran underneath my son's house also and Roy advised that this was not a safe house to live in or sleep in, yet my daughter's house was completely fine. Roy demonstrated to me the difference between the rhythms of the earth's natural current and the disrupting rhythms and disturbed current delivered to our bodies when sleeping in our bed. I stood barefoot in the garden and Roy measured the current which my body was receiving. I then lay on our bed and Roy again measured the current — the difference in the readings was astonishing! He then measured the current delivered to my body again after placing an earthing sheet, especially designed by Roy, under my feet on the bed which meant that I was earthed to the same rhythm as when I stood barefoot in the garden.

Roy explained that the electrical appliances left on all night and mobile phones would be interfering with the earth's current. We have a mobile phone mast on our land, not too far away from the house, and I was unsure if that was causing disturbance and radiation. Roy measured the disturbance from the mast and from all of our mobile phones and a cordless land line phone. It proved that the cordless land line phone was actually causing more disturbance than the mobile phone mast and the mobile phones so I threw it away and replaced it with a Siemens Gigaset S685 which Roy assured me was much better and safer than the one I had.

I bought earthing sheets for all of the beds and bought a gigantic one to put under the carpet in my son's house downstairs. I also bought a RadiTech (a multi–wave oscillator which eradicates electro–magnetic stress) and placed that in the living room underneath the main bedroom. I felt the difference immediately with the use of the earthing sheet and slept much better; Joe also slept better. I knew that I had to try and move Joe into another bedroom which would be better to sleep in so I created the perfect bedroom; no springs in the bed, earthing sheet, no electrical appliances and a blackout blind. I slept like a dream in it and still do now, but Joe never felt comfortable in there, preferring to suffer broken sleep and impaired health for his television and cameras.

Included with kind permission from Roy Riggs

Detox Electrolysis Footbath

There is much controversy about whether this actually achieves its objective, but the theory is as follows;

An electrical charge is passed between two electrodes which release negative ions into a small foot bath with water and salt added. The negative ions resonate with the body through the soles of the feet and bind to and neutralise positively charged toxins in the body. The toxins and other pollutants are then eliminated through the skin, kidneys, lungs and gut. The detox footbath helps to eliminate acids, uric acid, waste products and damaging substances rapidly and thoroughly leaving cells in the body electrically revitalised and the body purified, leading to a strengthened immune system and improved sleep quality.

The detox footbath can be used every other day. Joe generally used it twice a week. After use, he felt relaxed and re–energised. Who can say whether this was due to the special footbath or the natural feeling of relaxation following a normal footbath? As long as it helped, that was all that mattered.

Iscador Mistletoe Therapy

We travelled to see a homeopathic doctor in Liverpool in the hope of trying the Mistletoe Therapy. Mistletoe Therapy is reported in many trials to help with the side–effects of chemotherapy and radiotherapy such as sickness, tiredness, weight loss, low immunity and pain relief. It has also been shown to slow down tumour growth. The treatment, an extract from the mistletoe plant, is usually given as a subcutaneous injection, but the doctor did not recommend the treatment for Joe. It was his opinion that Joe's cancer was too advanced for the Mistletoe Therapy to have any worthwhile effect. Instead we were given the treatment in a liquid form to be taken orally.

I cannot say that we saw any visible improvements with the treatment but this would be in line with the doctor's opinion. There are many testimonies on the internet, however, which report positive responses.

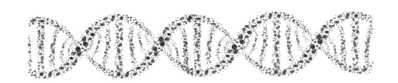

12 — And So The Story Ends

Thoughts of the Day

The thoughts which go through your head during the hard times make strange reading. The need to maintain normality as if the world couldn't suddenly end tomorrow rings through these extracts as I read them again. I've included them in the hope that some small emotion or thought might help someone to know that it's okay to feel sad, scared, hopeful and hopeless, and that it's all part of the journey which we share in our fight.

Friday 13ᵗʰ August 2010

On another trip to London we met up with Professor Oliver in the Oyster Bar in Harrods to discuss treatments over a few oysters and a glass of wine. We chatted about our meeting earlier with a specialist surgeon regarding Joe's osteonecrosis of the jaw. It was obvious that nothing could be done about this apart from keeping it clean, administering antibiotics and painkillers. We discussed trying to reduce the morphine dose if possible. I had read on the train on the way down how morphine can stimulate angiogenesis (new blood vessel growth that feeds rapidly growing tumours), activate a tumour cell survival signal and inhibit apoptosis. Morphine can also impair immune functions. Prof agreed, but also explained that it is extremely stressful to the body to be in pain and under constant suffering and misery, so being comfortable is an important thing. It was all about finding a happy medium.

Prof and I congratulated each other again on another result. The PSA was coming down, having fallen from 52 to 34.49 in one week — success again! Prof glanced at all of my shopping bags and smiled — I had quickly managed a little shopping in between appointments. We discussed the current protocol — docetaxel and bevacizumab — which seemed to be working well. I enquired how long we might keep using this treatment second time around. Prof explained that, as it was a low dose weekly, it should be effective for longer than before, which had been a good five months, but with any cancer prognosis it is virtually impossible to give an accurate period of effectiveness. Unfortunately, at this stage the alternative medicine can only add to the effect of the drugs and help to alleviate the symptoms. The cancer has become too aggressive.

Joe had been telling Prof that he had left school at twelve years of age with only one pair of trousers. Prof was excited — you must write a book — you must write all this down — our fight to survive cancer, a journey to the end with no stone unturned. Prof continued to tell us of his current works with underprivileged schools, giving children without opportunity the chance to enjoy some things in life. He said that too much importance is placed on higher education nowadays and, although the frequency of success may be greater after higher education, people can succeed without it. He said that Joe was an example of this type of success.

As an extreme example of this experience he described a chance encounter during a trip to South Africa when he met up with an African who, though not allowed to play golf in the Apartheid era, had been a caddy for a long period of his life and had learnt so well that his handicap was two. He was injured in a road accident and on crutches for six months, lost his job, his house and his wife. He was making a living by watching people's cars in unsafe areas of South Africa, living in an illegal squat under plastic sheets. He had only one shoe because the other one had been stolen whilst he was on crutches and he walked with a limp. He came towards Prof's car to offer to look after it and was practicing his golf swing. Prof then learnt that the man had forty children who he was teaching to play golf with cast–offs donated by his former colleagues. They all lived in the same squatter camps in South Africa.

Prof's interest was aroused and the first email he opened when he returned home was from someone who had helped him found the Orchid Cancer Research charity (see *www.orchid-cancer.org. uk*) that supported his work. Knowing of Prof's work on the use of exercise in both preventing cancer and slowing growth after diagnosis, he had news about a new form of 'Eco 20/20 style' golf played with special tennis balls and Velcro posts on any surface that his son, an ex–golf pro, had begun to use called SNAG — Starting New At Golf (*see www.snageurope.com/*) — to teach golf in under-privileged schools in the UK. Because of his experience in South

Africa, Prof immediately saw the potential to use this system as the basis for Orchid's school education programme for prevention of cancer (*see www.orchid-cancer.org.uk/738/Sport-&-Education*).

Having moved the conversation away from the cancer, Prof was curious to know more about Joe. How had Joe got his first break? From that very day, I thought about writing my book. Joe encouraged me and wanted me to write it. It is a tribute to Joe, a truly wonderful man.

Tuesday 31st August 2010

After another day in the London Clinic, here I am sat on the train back to Yorkshire. All is going well. The PSA has really come down now to 15 from 52 five weeks ago. The haemoglobin is the only problem now as that is coming down also and is now at 10.2. Apparently, this is the effect of the chemotherapy. I can tell by Joe's breathing as he is breathing more heavily which happened the last time that it came down to 9 when he had to have a blood transfusion which worked well and he was able to have more chemotherapy.

This last week Joe has had increasing pain in his jaw. I had to increase the base line morphine when I found that one night he drank almost 150ml of oral morphine. Today we met with Prof as we are trying to understand why the pain is so bad. Prof believes that maybe there is some cancer in the jaw area now as there has been a lot of inflammation which attracts the cancer. We have a couple of options; if the jaw settles after the chemotherapy treatment today then that is an indication that there may be some cancer in the area of the jaw and Prof will see about a small dose of radiation being administered to the area which may settle things down. He will also see about the possibilities of extracting the tooth as this probably harbours a significant amount of bacteria and infection underneath it. We are unsure as to whether the cranio–maxillofacial specialist will want to remove the tooth as there is already osteonecrosis of the jaw. This problem is still very new to the medical world and sometimes it is better to leave extraction well alone for fear of breaking part of the jaw bone off. Prof suggested using morphine patches, applied every three days, as these will release a constant level dose of morphine and may be a better way of administering it for maintaining pain relief throughout the night.

I popped into my favourite shop whilst in London, the whole foods store on Kensington High Street, full of my favourite organic foods and products: paraben free shampoo, conditioner, body lotions and toothpaste without sodium lauryl sulphate which are a lot less toxic for the body.

22nd September 2010

The waves fight violently amongst themselves today, hurling huge volcanoes of white mist into the turbulent air. All I can see is white. We are sailing on our yacht from the South of France to Genoa where we plan to leave the boat — maybe for the winter, maybe forever. It would be a miracle of miracles if Joe lasts to make another summer, but who knows, for miracles keep happening.

He now weighs thirteen stone, down from sixteen and a half. His legs and arms, once so strong and firm, are so thin and weak that he struggles to climb any stairs and sometimes has to go up on all fours. Thankfully his will remains strong, his desire to fight and stay alive strong. He continues to set himself new challenges.

He has been sick every morning this last week and eaten very little for days. I will have to stop some of the tablets from America. It often happens that I have to stop some tablets and then restart them when he gets a little stronger, starts to eat again and is no longer being sick.

I always wanted to be a doctor. Maybe this is God's way of giving me my opportunity to be one in a small way, caring for Joe. The doctors everywhere are amazed at how dedicated and determined I have been and how I make decisions just as they would. A couple of doctors at the clinic in London have praised me for my work and I know that Professor Oliver has always been excited when I come along with yet another alternative treatment or medicine to add to his conventional medicine. The doctors say that Joe is lucky to have his own personal doctor 24/7 — everyone would love one of those.

I also spent years looking after my son who had extremely bad asthma from the age of six weeks to about seven years. I needed to sit with him for four hours every day giving him a nebuliser (a delivery device which created a mist of medicine which went over the mouth and nose to help him breath). He then went on to have fits too. Fortunately these were only febrile convulsions and he grew out of these when he was four years old. I found that when I put him on special diets — no sugar, no dairy, no processed foods — that his asthma got much, much better. I didn't know as much then as I know now about how important diet is for the health.

27ᵗʰ September 2010

What a morning! I thought that we would save money by pre-booking first class rail tickets, but then Joe forgot the credit card which we had used to book them. Jenna came to the rescue with a last minute dash to bring the card and we made our pre-booked tickets. Joe was a little forgetful this morning. It would not register that the train was at 9.05 even though I told him three times. Never mind, at least he says that he feels good, so that's all that matters. He has regained his appetite after two weeks of treatment and a few days of rest from the tablets. Yesterday he was like hungry Horace eating everything. He said that he was starving and got up for more food at 3am — a definite improvement.

12ᵗʰ October 2010

The last couple of weeks Joe has not been himself. He has been very quiet, not wanting to talk. I looked at his blood under the microscope and was shocked to see how horrendous it looked with big, white puddles showing massive free radical damage to the cells. Joe was extremely alarmed by this. A good thing came out of it though as he decided that he is going to take all of my alternative medicines again to try to improve things.

I also just received results back from some urine tests which I sent to America. I sent a sample of both mine and Joe's urine just to see what the difference in results would be. It was remarkable. Joe's urine showed fatty acid oxidation, glucose oxidation, renal ammonia loading, impaired valine metabolism (valine is an amino acid), chronic low total body glutathione, intestinal bacteria overgrowth and clostridial species (anaerobes that cause disease in humans). All of this against mine which showed only that I had undergone a severe detox. This now gives me very good ammunition to make Joe take my supplements.

I managed to get a night away alone this last weekend to give me a bit of time with my daughter as to be honest most of my time is spent with Joe. It was a really nice break, but drank too much and ended up crying which is usual when I drink too much. I suppose I need to let my emotions out from time to time as I mostly feel sad when I have to see Joe so miserable every day and suffering. Chemotherapy is very harsh and it is slowly killing him, but at the same time keeping him alive. I wish that I could cry and tell him how sorry I feel for him and how much I love him, but I can't. I have to be strong for him.

14<u>th</u> October 2010

I find it so difficult to put pen to paper to write how I feel. I am sitting on a flight to the Bahamas. Thank you, Lord, for helping me to get here. It's been a family holiday planned six weeks ago. We shall meet a one hundred and ten foot boat with four crew members for eight nights.

Last night I never thought I would get here. Joe has been very weak since his last treatment. He has been in bed for two and a half days hardly eating anything. I made up a protein drink made with soya milk and a supplement called Spiru–tein which has many minerals, vitamins and amino acids and, when he cannot face food, he can usually manage one of these. This is all that he has eaten all week, plus electrolyte drinks. He has had diarrhoea for a whole week so I had to regularly give him electrolyte drinks otherwise his blood pressure would go really low.

We arrived at the hotel in London last night. Joe was tired and wanted to get to the room and lay down. He was cold and his teeth were chattering so I sent him to the room alone while I continued with the check in. What a mistake! He went to the wrong floor and could not find where he should be. He was calling for me to help him. He could not control his bowels. I eventually left the check in and went to find him with assistance. He had lost so much fluid; he was so embarrassed. Fortunately they had a room close by where we could go to get him cleaned up. I can still see his little face, helpless, confused, shivering, stood at the end of the corridor. I got him into bed and covered him with blankets and dressing gowns.

Coincidentally, Prof called me just at that moment to see how things were going. When I told him what had happened he wanted to admit Joe to hospital, but I knew that Joe would hate that and I felt that I had everything under control. Prof said that he wanted to admit him in the morning just to check him over and give him some fluids. I agreed. But after about an hour Joe started to come round and would have none of it. He said that he was fine and would be okay to go away. Prof decided that he would call by the hotel early in the morning instead to check him over. He called me at 6.30am to say that he was on his way. We all went for breakfast, Joe saying that he was feeling much better. He did eat a little, whether because he wanted it or just to convince Prof that he was okay, I don't know. Prof and I agreed that he would be okay to travel. Prof brought along a letter that we could take with us which stated Joe's current medication and his medical history just in case we had an emergency abroad. Yippee, off we go to the sunshine for some vitamin D. I think that the sunshine has helped to keep Joe going all these years.

Here now in the Bahamas, the sunshine seems to be cheering him up. He is still not eating much but he is improving every day. When we arrived, his elbow looked rather infected and puss was coming out of it. I looked on the internet for alternative cures and decided to try crushed garlic directly on to the open wound. I left it for three hours and then put antibiotic cream on it that evening. I started him on a high dose of Allitech strong allicin, garlic capsules available from Dulwich Health *(www.dulwichhealth.co.uk)*, and three days later his elbow is now as good as new. It is said that these capsules and liquid are the best known cure for MRSA.

Joe's jaw is growing bone now underneath. I contacted the cranio–maxillofacial specialist about this and was told that this is not unusual. I spoke to Dr Jacobs at the Cancer Clinic today who is always so positive and gives me such inspiration. She told me about an injection that is proving successful in treating osteonecrosis of the jaw. Apparently it encourages new bone growth. After telling Joe about this he seemed much happier — his jaw has been a real problem for him.

Well, we are nearing the end of our holiday now. It has gone so quickly. The Bahamas are truly an unspoilt paradise when visited on a boat. The sea is crystal clear with lots of fish and natural coral. Lurking are many sharks and stingrays which can be quite scary, but everyone says that the sharks don't bother you as they are only nurse sharks.

We saw the weirdest thing on one of the islands. A small, single engine seaplane had landed in the sea close to the beach where wild pigs live. Visitors would come to this small island and feed the pigs. The man flying the aircraft said that he had flown all the way from Fort Lauderdale just to feed them. He had a video camera set up on the wing and was recording himself feeding the wild pigs. They were jumping up onto the wing, snapping at the plates of food and loaves of bread which he had brought for them and then they tried to bite his leg! What a character he was! We went back to our boat to get food for the pigs and when we returned we heard the plane engines and off he went into the horizon.

We also visited the island where they filmed the movie 'Blow'. It's now an island with many derelict buildings, but people still live there. Small planes still land there — we saw three coming and going in one day. A small boat would arrive when the aeroplane landed and would leave as the plane took off. Somehow it was quite a spooky little island.

Well, we managed to get Joe on a jet ski out in the sun and even trying to do a little fishing. He was resurrected again! Although now I can beat him at arm wrestling, such a strong fit man before and now so weak. Exercise was never his passion and he stopped exercising probably this time last year when he started to become weak with the chemotherapy. Now he is as weak as a kitten. Thankfully, he is eating again now, so with some good nutritious food we should be able to build him back up.

I feel like Joe's illness is my battle, my enemy because I am the only one strong enough to fight it for him. Would I be like this if it happened to me? I woke at 5am; well, Joe woke me. Always the same question in my head — what can we do next? There are other treatments out there but I must research them more. I cannot make the wrong decisions. We are waiting for the new drug abiraterone to come out — it can't be long now, early next year I think. I am going to keep him alive until then — well I am going to try my best. I shall research more about Jetvana, a new chemo drug for advanced prostate cancer. It is still new and much less tried than the docetaxel. I am unsure. I will look into this more.

November 3ʳᵈ 2010

I lay on the bed with Joe, an evening ritual. Sadly, I can no longer sleep in the same bed and haven't for about a year. I simply can't rest there, but I always try to spend an hour cuddled up to him. Savouring the warmth of him, I wanted to see his lovely face. Tears streamed down his face; he was crying.

'Don't cry darling, don't cry,' I whispered. I sobbed with him. Then I changed my mind and breathed quietly, 'You cry darling if you want to cry. Don't hold everything inside, you cry.' Then he let everything out. He cried and cried so loudly, the deep emotion tearing free from its chains.

'I can't do anything,' he sobbed. 'What's the point? All I do is sleep. What's the point in carrying on.'

'You're going nowhere,' I whispered, 'you are not giving in. Anyway you can't give in,' I replied in an attempt to lighten him, 'because we're going to the Maldives for Christmas and New Year. You have to take me there.'

I didn't really mean this — I didn't care where we were as long as we were together — but I knew that looking forward to his trips kept him going because he enjoyed them so much. I had to pretend to be cold-hearted and selfish because that kept him stronger. I felt so bad, so cruel, when really I just wanted to hold him and give in too, but I knew that I couldn't.

It's getting very hard for me to see my strong husband so weak. He is slowly dying in front of me. What can I do now to save him? His PSA is coming down every week, but I sense that something is wrong. I've learnt how to listen to his cancer, my constant companion.

Joe thinks that he will die when he is sixty. He predicted this at the same time as correctly predicting that our son would be born on his fortieth birthday.

'I will be back tomorrow to have my son,' I said to the specialist on the 17th of November. 'My husband told me to tell you.'

'I don't think so,' laughed the specialist, as this would mean that my baby would be three weeks premature. 'I will see you when I return from my holidays!' He could hardly believe it when I gave birth to Jordan the next day, as predicted, on Joe's fortieth birthday.

I think that he is giving in as he believes that he will be right again.

I should go away at the weekend for two nights to visit my friend in Norway but the thought of having to leave him is killing me.

'I don't really want to leave you, darling,' I tell him. 'I feel so bad, will you be okay?' Of course he said yes and that he would be fine, don't worry.

The kids agreed to do a day each taking good care of him. I needed a break, but felt so guilty and neglectful to go. I left all of his tablets labelled out on a pin board.

It was a rewarding break, a chance to get my strength back to be able to fight for him, but I was sad. I shall never leave him again. We met back up together in London last night. He was really pleased to see me, as though he could relax again now that I was back by his side.

The Cancer Clinic wanted another scan to see what was happening, a PET scan. We went early to the hospital in London and Professor Oliver's secretary carried out a blood test to send off to America (as we could not find any hospital, whether private or not, who could carry out CTC tests) to check the CTCs . She took another normal blood sample to check the haemoglobin level and PSA to see if there was any indication as to why he was sleeping so much. They performed the PET scan, after which he looked exhausted. We then went for some food which left him feeling terribly sick.

Whilst Joe was having his scan, I popped off for breast thermography. It's a way of looking at the breast to look for abnormalities, mainly in the lymph. I was told that I had a backup of gristle in the lymph area under my arm and that this could lead to breast disease. The doctor suggested a lymphatic drainage treatment straight away which she carried out there and then. She then repeated the breast thermography and it showed results of lymph waste being moved immediately. She recommended a follow-up and more lymphatic treatment. She added that she would post the results to America for an expert opinion and would send me the results. It's been two years now since I had my breasts examined. I am neglecting myself as I am so busy with Joe — I was having ultrasound twice a year and a mammogram at least once a year, both precautionary. After reading so much about the negative effects of too many mammograms I have decided not to have as many, and I have decided to try breast thermography along with ultrasound as an alternative. We will see how this goes.

We return now on the train. Joe is sleeping, yet again. I watch him every second, hoping and praying that he will be okay.

November 11th 2010

The results have arrived from America and they are not good. Joe will need to have more chemotherapy soon otherwise I am sure that he will be sick and unable to travel at Christmas. It now appears that the lump in his jaw, close to the osteonecrosis, could be a small cancerous growth.

I can't tell Joe the terrible news. I obviously have to tell him something — I can't lie.

'Darling, it doesn't look great,' is the best that I could do. There may be some concern about his liver and maybe one lymph node. His stomach is clear though, and his lungs and his brain, so that's great. To me this means that we have a fighting chance, at least for a few months.

'I think you will have to have some more treatment, darling, some more chemo and some radiotherapy to the jaw,' I told him as unconcernedly as I could manage.

'What will happen if I don't have it, will I die?'

'Probably.' I have to tell him the truth.

'Oh, it's nearly the end,' he says.

'Don't be negative now. We have never been negative. Don't start now, think positive. We have a lovely trip to look forward to at Christmas, to the Maldives. You have to take me there.' He keeps saying now that it's nearly the end, it's getting close. Is he saying it because he doesn't want it or because he's tired of fighting?

Again I have been researching on the internet about his symptoms — hoarse voice, numbness in the jaw, a lot of phlegm in the throat — all signs of head and neck cancers. I search metastatic liver cancer which highlights the fact that there is nothing more that medicine can do, and so the patient is dying. How do I deal with this? How patient's wishes differ! Some patients end their life in denial, without finishing things off, and this is their way of coping with the prospect of death. This is Joe. He has finalised many things, but he will never let his business go — this will go with him. If we manage to continue it when he has gone, then that would be marvellous. If we don't, then he will never know. This is his baby, the only thing that he has left to keep him going — apart from us of course. My heart sinks, I sob alone. Just as quickly I slap myself. No, I will not be negative, I never have been. I will continue just as if everything is the same.

The evening draws in, it's late. Every day is very stressful. Besides the fear of Joe dying and the continued struggle to stay one step ahead of his cancer, I am trying to learn as much as I can about the business, about tax affairs, in readiness for the inevitable. I have learnt much this last year. I need to know how to carry things on in case something should happen to Joe. He has the answers for everyone. He is so clever. We all look to him to answer our questions: my son, my daughter, his workforce and me. We all admire him so much for what he has achieved.

Over the last few days I can see that Joe is thinking a lot. He is quiet, sleeping a lot too. The lump on his jaw is getting bigger. I am not sure if it is an abscess as well as a cancerous lump as it looks to have a head on it. He is in constant pain now, although relieved somewhat by the morphine. He saw a programme on television about how people with cancer are using cannabis for pain relief and relaxation and he decided that he was going to try it. What could I say? Nothing. His friend brought him some but without tobacco in so that, apparently, he would not get addicted. A positive effect was that it gave him an incredible appetite. One day he had eaten hardly anything. Then he had some 'happy backy' cannabis and he never stopped eating for the rest of the day. Well, they do say it gives you the munchies and it relaxed him somewhat. He uses it now if he does not feel like eating. He says that it doesn't really relieve the pain, well not for him, but it has other benefits. However, I wasn't impressed when I went into the bedroom and smelt it in the cupboard. I tried to be angry. My son came into the bedroom and asked if someone had been smoking in there.

'Yes, your mother,' he laughed. We all had a chuckle. I can't get angry with him, although it would have been easy to be angry because cannabis was a very sore subject for us all. My son went through years of smoking it, unbeknown to us, and by the time that we found out he was completely addicted. He had become a little monster and his mood swings were uncontrollable. He said unforgivable things to all of the family. He isolated himself from us and never came on any holidays. As a last resort we had to make him leave his house, which was next to ours on our large farm, and we sacked him from his job. In broad Yorkshire terms we had to 'throw him out' and let him learn about the real world. He blamed his father's diagnosis for starting to smoke it in the beginning. My son has always found it extremely hard to deal with his dad's illness, more so than anyone. Cannabis was probably his way of blotting out the reality. Eventually, and thankfully, my son turned a corner, found himself a lovely girlfriend and stopped smoking cannabis. He is now a different young man. I cannot believe that now I have his father smoking cannabis, albeit for very different reasons — or are they?

<u>14<u>th</u> November 2010</u>

Well, we are finally here on the plane to the Turcs and Caicus Islands to celebrate my son's twenty–first birthday. Joe's prediction, that he will die when he is sixty, will not come true. We never seriously thought that we would make that one, yet he is going to make sixty–

one. His jaw is really swollen from the flight. We arrive at the boat, the same boat as in the Bahamas. It's amazing — 'Da Bubba' — named after the owner's pet dog. The crew is very welcoming and it's great to be back on board.

The following morning Joe wakes up early in pain with his jaw. He asks for painkillers. Later in the day puss weeps from out of the jaw and it looks like it is just an abscess or boil there. The swelling has gone down considerably now following the flow of puss. Joe is kind of relieved — maybe it's not cancer in his jaw after all.

18th November 2010

Six years from the diagnosis and my son's twenty–first birthday and Joe's sixty–first birthday. It is an achievement for us to get him here. We all enjoy a relaxed birthday celebration together. Deep down we all know that it will be the last one. Joe must have had the cancer for a few years prior to diagnosis as it had already spread to his bones. Maybe he has had it for ten years or more now, who knows? It certainly went undiagnosed for nearly a year prior to the diagnosis.

19th November 2010

I called the Cancer Clinic today to see if they have received the scan results. I talked to Dr Jacobs who tells me not to continue with any of the current treatments as they are completely wrong now as the cancer has changed its course — the current treatment will no longer work. No wonder Joe was so ill after his last lot of treatment. Maybe we should have gone back to the Cancer Clinic before going away. In any case, Dr Jacobs will give Joe a new treatment protocol. They are so advanced and knowledgeable at the Cancer Clinic that they generally know from experience what course to follow if something fails.

29th November 2010

Last Monday we arrived at the clinic in London. I was desperate to start Joe on the new treatment which the Cancer Clinic had recommended. Prof arrived to meet us there and miraculously he had organised everything. I could not believe that Joe was to get all of the new treatments there and then, except for one tablet, vorinostat, which the clinic in London could not get. I would have to contact the Cancer Clinic and see if I could get that through them.

He had blood tests first which more or less pointed to the fact that the Cancer Clinic was right in their diagnosis, signalled by the PSA not rising a great deal, but Joe's health deteriorating. We would have to use different blood tests now to assess the development of the cancer. Prof said that Joe would have to rest.

We are so lucky to have found Prof. In the medical profession you meet good and bad, some specialists really speak down to you, and some GPs I have found to be in another world. I have found that having educated myself about cancer and disease it has helped me both in dealing with the doctors and in helping to keep Joe as well as possible.

It's a week now since starting the new treatment and Joe has been in pain all week. I have had to increase the morphine and give more steroids every day. Gosh, maybe it's not working. What shall I do? I will meet Prof at the clinic in London and get the bloods done and see from there.

It's a real strain on me every day having to hear him screaming with pain. He looks so weak. I reflect his strain on my own face. I feel like the end is near, I'm afraid. Will he make Christmas? I really don't know.

After seeing Prof earlier today, I feel reassured that things aren't so bad. Bone pain can be experienced at the beginning of a new treatment protocol until the body gets used to the drugs, so we must persevere. We discussed the treatments to help build and protect the bone — teriparatide and denosumab. Prof was very apprehensive about giving Joe these as he did not want to bombard him with too many different and potentially counterindicative drugs. He was also very wary about any drugs which affected the bone anywhere in the body following the osteonecrosis, but he agreed in the end to try teriparatide. This will be in the form of a subcutaneous injection given daily, and then denosumab next week if the bone pain does not subside — a result again! I asked Prof how long steroids will work if all else fails — will we get to the Maldives for Christmas?

'Oh yes,' he said, 'he can survive for six weeks on steroids.' They call it the honeymoon period, so that if the treatment did fail then at least he will get Christmas pain free and in the sunshine, hopefully with his family.

The new tablet, vorinostat, finally arrived from America. We started on them straight away on Friday. Disturbingly, by the evening Joe was feeling red hot. He had been lying in bed all day, literally, saying that he had nothing to do. Concerned, I read what could be expected as a side–effect of the drug and sure enough there was 'fever' followed by the advice to contact your doctor if you experience any of the said side–effects. I called the doctor on call at the Cancer Clinic who told me to check over Joe's body to see if anything looked unusual. I pulled the covers back so that I could give him a quick wash down with some cool flannels and investigate as I had been asked. His body was red in places, particularly his left leg which was also very inflamed, together with his foot. The doctor told me to immediately call the emergency services and have them check him out. I called the ambulance service, panicking and stressed, who came quickly, the medics advising that they suspected, as did I, deep vein thrombosis. They suggested that Joe should go to the hospital in the ambulance but he didn't want to go! He was laughing and said that he was fine. Thankfully, after some persuasion, my daughter and I got him into the ambulance. We followed close behind. Jenna and I sat for hours in the hospital. Joe's blood pressure was high — 147 over 97. The diagnosis was that he definitely had deep vein thrombosis so they gave him a blood thinning injection and a heart scan. His heart seemed to be pumping well. We were told to return twenty four hours later for another injection which had to be administered every twenty four hours for up to six months and we were advised to stop all treatment until the problem was under control.

My heart sank because now there was one more problem to add to everything else. This would now probably mean that we would have to stop the new tablet vorinostat as it is contraindicated (not advisable to be used at the same time as another specific substance) with blood thinners and its possible side–effects include blood clots. Dr Jacobs was of the opinion that it was just coincidental that this had occurred after only taking one vorinostat. Dr Fredericks recommended that we did not continue with it as a precaution. This meant that we probably would not be able to achieve the results which we had hoped for with the new treatment protocol.

I have now spoken to Dr Jacobs and Professor Oliver. In their opinion it seems we will be able to restart all treatment apart from vorinostat, the new tablet, as that is contraindicated to blood thinners. He will have to have a daily injection of enoxaparin sodium, which I will have to administer as it is very difficult to keep the same levels of blood with oral tablets and they are contraindicated to more things.

I have heard of deep vein thrombosis but here we are now faced with it. Joe is becoming less and less active by the day and maybe if he had been more active then he might not have the problem. We are on our way to London now to have the next chemo and hopefully to collect some blood–thinning injections.

Some time in January 2011

Well we made it to the New Year 2011, returning now from the Maldives. We both wanted this so much, for the family to spend the Christmas and New Year together. It was a sort of ritual and cancer wasn't going to spoil it — I know that he did it for me and the children, but it gave him the will to go on.

Joe has changed and I could see over the holiday how frustrated he seems. He is so weak — he can no longer lift his legs to climb up a high step. He couldn't go on any fishing trips for fear that he would not be able to get back off the boat, apart from one time. He couldn't fish as he was so weak, and when he got off the boat he fell backwards. Luckily someone caught him, but he still managed to cut open his toe and leg. This was his second accident as, when he first arrived, he managed to hook himself in the lip with a fishing hook from a rod which someone had bought him for Christmas whilst he was removing the wrapping with his teeth. Fortunately, the doctor had anaesthetic and managed to do a small cut to the lip to remove it.

At the beginning of the trip Joe was like a monster. He was so horrible to me, coming back with sarcastic comments to everything that I said until, in the end, I snapped and said that's enough. He changed after that and became a little nicer.

'I keep thinking you are to blame for all my pain,' he said. 'I keep blaming you for all this suffering.' I don't understand why, and neither did he. He said he didn't really enjoy the trip.

'You are all enjoying things and I cannot enjoy anything but the sun,' he complained. He is becoming very negative and can only say bad things about people all day.

The first week of the holiday he was in pain with his back. I was giving him 4mg of dexamethasone steroid tablets but this was not controlling it. I decided to up the steroids to 12mg to try and get rid of the pain and give him some comfort. Fortunately, this worked and he seemed better. It seems that I need to use the steroids more frequently now to control the pain.

It is three weeks now since his last injection of **bortezomib**. I can see that the cancer is back with a vengeance. He has a lot of mucous in his throat, especially in the morning, and he is very weak. I had to have wheelchair assistance throughout the airport and to get him on and off the plane. He cannot even open a lid any more. I can smell the cancer coming back. Some days he smells like a piece of raw meat — every time it starts to come back I can smell it.

He is beginning to worry now and he thinks his life is coming to the end. I am sure it is, but I will not let these thoughts enter into my head. I will never believe that he is dying even though it is more apparent now than ever.

He will restart his treatment on Monday and I hope that we have not given him too long a break in between to allow the cancer to become too strong. Was this going to be our last trip ever?

We returned from the Maldives on the 2nd of January. On the 3rd January Joe was due his treatment which was the new protocol which was working quite well before Christmas.

To be honest, I don't think we should have travelled so far to the Maldives, but Joe wanted to. He wanted to carry on life as normally as possible. The long flights always put an incredible strain on his body and he would sometimes have bouts of pain during or after them. Flying long haul exposes the body to a lot of radiation. We probably should not have broken the treatment protocol either — he carried on taking all of his tablets except vorinostat but stopped the bortezomib injection — but I really do not think that Joe would have been strong enough to take another dose over the Christmas period, he was too weak. Prof said that the cancer does not go on holiday. He was right; the cancer did not have a rest, it carried on multiplying.

Joe had the treatment and he decided that he wanted to drive around all of the demolition jobs that he had. He told me to get a campervan so that we could drive and stay in the van at night which wasn't very practical but I agreed. He wanted Jenna and the site manager to come to London and go with us. It seemed like a last stand! Joe was so determined.

We travelled to Bridgewater, then to Wales in search of a piece of land in Saron that we own. When we arrived there it was drawing dark. We drove round and round the area where we thought the land was, but in the end it was too dark and we couldn't see it. We travelled then to Cardiff and stayed in a hotel overnight. When we got into the hotel room Joe was exhausted. Tears trickled down his face, but all that I could do to help was hug him.

'You are exhausted darling,' I whispered. He didn't want to eat anything. I comforted him, saying, 'Just try and have a sleep darling and you might feel better.' I went to the bar to let him rest and to have a glass of wine with Jenna and the site manager. I went back after a short while and he seemed a little brighter. We ordered food from room service, but he didn't eat anything.

The following day Joe seemed a bit better. We headed off to Cardiff, then up to Nantwich and then to Mexborough. He went and saw all of his jobs and all of his men, some who had worked for him for thirty years.

We arrived home that evening, and again he went to work the next day. By this time, it was evident that he was really weakening. He could hardly climb up the stairs and he would stand at the bottom and will himself to climb them on all fours. On Saturday I helped him to get ready to go to the jobs with the site manager and Jenna. I had to dress him as he couldn't even put on his own trousers or socks. He slid down the stairs on his bottom. He sat on the sofa waiting for the site manager to arrive but, when he did, Joe couldn't get up off the sofa. He got down on the floor.

'Don't let him see me,' he said. I couldn't lift him up, he was too heavy, so I fetched a walking stick and he used it to will himself to his feet.

I knew that soon he would not be able to get up the stairs at all, so I ordered a stair–lift which was due to be fitted on the 11th January, but there was some delay and it was never installed.

On the Saturday whilst Joe was out I went and bought a wheelchair. He couldn't manage any longer and I needed to try to make it easier for him. When Joe got back I told him.

'I don't need a wheelchair,' he growled, thought about it and said, 'bring it in then, let's have a look.' I brought it into the living room for him to see. He got in it.

'It's no good,' he shouted. 'I can't push myself. It doesn't have big wheels.' I told him that I'd push him.

'Well, what happens if you leave me on a hill and I can't stop myself?' he half joked.

'Silly, I'm not likely to do that.'

'Well, what happens when we go to Las Vegas and you go off shopping and leave me somewhere or I want to go look somewhere else by myself?'

'Well, I'll buy another with big wheels, and you can decide which one we take with us wherever we are going.' Determined to the end.

We were due to do our usual trip to London on Monday for treatment but Joe said he did not want to go.

'You have to go, darling, I have organised everything. I will take the wheelchair. I have organised the train. They will put a ramp onto the platform so I can wheel you on and I have arranged a mini-van to collect us at the station and take us to the hospital.' He did not want any of it. He did not want to go in the wheelchair. He organised a driver instead and the driver drove him to the clinic in London.

Joe had his blood taken. His haemoglobin level was quite low, so they decided that they would give him three units of blood. This was going to take some time and they advised that we would have to stay overnight so that they could start to administer the blood early the next morning. They gave him one unit later that day and he seemed fine.

They started to give Joe the blood early the next morning. After a short time Joe became extremely distressed and in a lot of pain. I thought it was maybe the cancer in the bones that was causing it, but he was in too much pain to tell me where it hurt. Eventually, the doctors realised that he had developed pneumothorax (a collection of gas or air in the lung or pleural space which causes all or part of the lung to collapse) and it was found that one lung had collapsed; Joe's oxygen levels were rapidly decreasing. They gave him oxygen and performed an emergency bedside operation to inflate the lung. This didn't work and soon after they had to perform another.

I rang my daughter and was obviously extremely distressed. She sensed it straight away and asked if I wanted her to come. I immediately replied yes! I called my son and told him that I thought he had better come and see his dad as he was really unwell. Joe was fighting to breathe.

We three stayed in the room with Joe all night, taking it in turns to monitor him and calling the nurse every three hours for more pain relief. I held his hand and kissed him continually. He kept asking why I was holding his hand.

'Because I want to,' I smiled, 'because I want to hold your hand, because I love you.' He smiled back.

A nurse had sat with us all day whilst he was being monitored before the children arrived.

'You know what she's doing don't you?' Joe asked.

'No.'

'She's counting the kisses.' Bless him! I wanted to cry but had to be strong. He never lost his sense of humour right to the end, nor his beautiful smile.

In the morning it was evident that his condition had severely worsened. I called the doctor who confirmed that there was an infection in the lungs, which had now progressed into pneumonia. They decided to transfer him to intensive care. We had a meeting with the head of the intensive care unit who said that they were going to try a special helmet on him which would help him to breathe until they could get antibiotics into him intravenously to treat the pneumonia. This worked for a while, but once they removed the helmet his oxygen level would deteriorate immediately and it was becoming lower and lower. Then they discovered that he had a large blood clot in his heart. His organs were giving up.

From time to time we would have to leave the intensive care room and wait in the waiting room whilst they performed their procedures, also turning him as his bottom was sore with being in the same position, and when we returned Joe said that he had overheard them saying that they couldn't operate, that there was nothing that they could do.

There was a nurse at the end of the bed who was in the process of doing observations.

'What's happening, did they say they can't operate? Why?' I demanded. I was hysterical. My daughter tried to calm me.

'Calm down mum. She doesn't know anything, calm down.'

We had yet another meeting with the head of the intensive care unit and his assistant. They explained that things were not going well and that the helmet which they had fitted was not enough and soon they would have to put him on a life support machine. This would mean giving him sufficient anaesthetic so that they could get the tube down his throat and he would probably die during the procedure. Did we want to do it? We had no need to discuss it — we knew what he would say if he could. We told them no, he would not want that, he had had enough.

We went back to Joe. He looked at me and tried to shake his head, his expression confirming our decision, that he'd had enough. We were kissing through the helmet so they removed it to let us have a proper hug and a kiss. Within thirty seconds he was hardly breathing so they had to quickly put the helmet back on. They tried another procedure to try and break down the blood clot in his heart which didn't work. They increased the morphine so he was not in any pain. I feared that he may die that evening as he was so weak.

My daughter, my son and I remained by his bedside. We lost him at 3am on the thirteenth of January 2011. I lost my love, my soul mate, my hero, the man of my dreams and my children lost their father. I must carry on now without him. I cried and cried, crying the tears that I'd held back for so long. I stayed with him for hours after. The hospital staff were very good and let me stay with him for as long as I needed so that I could say goodbye. One last goodbye.

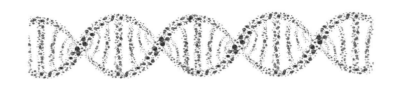

13 — Life After Joe

I found myself in Austria, finally putting pen to paper again, five months on from the death of my wonderful husband Joseph. How did I get there?

A friend recommended the clinic.

'Oh, don't you go to the Mayr Clinic darling?' she asked. 'My boss goes twice a year — it's meant to be fabulous.' Ok I thought, a hotel on a lake, beautiful setting, sounds like an ideal spot to write my book. That's all I knew.

This is now my third trip to Austria. The clinic turned out to be everything that I needed and remains so; no distractions by long meal times with huge meals, no alcohol and, most importantly, just peace and tranquility. Although there are many guests, the place is so big that it never seems crowded and there is plenty of room to find your own piece of space to be alone. This time, however, I am not alone. My sister has accompanied me as we are working together on finalising this book for Joe.

When I first came, five months after Joe's death, I was in a terrible place. I was alone for the first time in twenty–eight years, without my soul mate, my best friend, my rock through thick and thin who never let me down. We rarely travelled separately and during the last seven years of Joe's life we became closer than we had ever been, joined in a personal two–man battle to keep him alive.

Almost two and a half years have passed by since Joe sadly lost his fight. I remember the day as though it was yesterday but block it from my mind as much as possible for self–preservation. The feelings which the memory brings with it are still too much to bear. It still seems like a bad dream from which I will wake and find that he is still with me. The love which I have for him has not dwindled in that time and my heart aches for him to hold me again, to tell me that everything will be okay. The tears fall less often, but the pain still feeds on my sadness. I think of him every hour of every day.

To survive I have kept myself very busy with work and sorting out the wonderful jigsaw puzzles which Joe left behind for me.

'When I have gone', he used to say, 'you will be moving all of those toyboys in and you will forget about me'. So, to keep me out of mischief, he left me much to solve with business and financial puzzles. The steep learning curve has certainly achieved his objective.

Other times he would say, 'come and cuddle me. You will be sorry when I have gone. When I have gone you will want me to come back'. How right he was. A part of me died with him, but I must carry on. I must finish this book for Joe and make sure that people are given the chance to learn from our journey so that we might help them to feel empowered to help themselves.

I enjoy helping others, using my knowledge to bring improved health and vigour to anyone that I meet, like the lady that I met on a plane recently. I gave her some advice and she was truly grateful. I know that if she makes those changes then she will prolong her fight against her cancer. Likewise, if my sister takes the advice which she is receiving this week then I know that she will get better.

Joe used to say 'you are only here once'. I don't believe that. I can still feel his presence with me in our home, still feel him trying to help me. How can such a strong character just disappear and leave this world forever? I feel sure that he is guiding me as he always did. He was always so quick, so streetwise both in life and business. Even his accountants and financial advisors struggled to keep up with him. Even without any learning he just had a knack for knowing the best thing to do, always one step ahead of everyone. He kept everything in his head, constantly thinking, plotting, planning, finding alternatives and constantly improving decisions. He would have his best ideas during the night when he couldn't sleep. I would wake up and he would say, 'I'm a genius! I have had another brainwave'. He was very creative and excellent at thinking outside the box.

Although Joe's passing left me with a great many headaches — puzzles as Joe liked to call them — I was very fortunate in that he left me in a comfortable financial position. This takes away many stresses which face wives who are left alone, but it does not bring him back. I would trade every single penny to have him back with me. It wasn't always the case that we were comfortable. Business has its ups and downs, its good times and bad. I remember one time when Joe had only one hundred pounds left in his pocket and the company was on the brink of going under. He told me that any day the banks might call in the loans and that we would also lose our home. He promptly left and headed for the shops, returning with two bottles of champagne and a huge smile on his face.

'What the heck!' he chuckled. 'Let's have a drink darling.' What a fighter. What a positive man. Memories such as these keep him close and make me smile.

Well, back to the Mayr Clinic. The commitment to come here once a year has been like a beacon in the distance, that if I can make it back for another year then I can be renewed and refreshed and start another year without him. There are several Mayr Clinics in Austria which offer a treatment known as the 'Mayr Cure'. Principally, the clinics are for detoxification and de-acidification of the body. The treatments are especially good for those suffering with allergies and digestive disorders, many of which may be unknown before visiting the clinic. It is also very therapeutic for those suffering from mental illnesses, providing a safe haven of support and solitude. Hunger is all part of the treatment, but it's a manageable hunger because you know that it is what your body needs. Guests are taught how to chew their food properly so that all of the enzymes can work on getting as many nutrients as possible from the food — especially interesting when it comes to chewing clear soup! It is the perfect place to give both the mind and body a rest, to renew vigour and positivity, to heal. I think that Joe would have liked it here.

Well, tomorrow I leave this refuge to return to the world without Joe. Next week our daughter will be married without her father to give her away. I wish with all my heart that her daddy could have seen his beautiful daughter become a wife. Yet another hurdle to overcome. Maybe one day they'll stop.

Joe's life may have ended but mine goes on. I hope that by adhering to a good, healthy, nutritious diet, with plenty of fruit and vegetables, no junk food, no processed foods, no dairy, little or no meat, various supplements (good quality only), good water, an alkaline diet, exercise, detoxing and most importantly a strong immune system (through all of this), that I will live a long and, most importantly, healthy life. I believe that the only barrier to this would be stress, which is harder to control. I have always been a 'party girl' and still am but I try to find a balance. I allow myself little treats; I drink alcohol on holidays and weekends, eat a small quantity of dark chocolate every day and drink one coffee a day. These are my indulgences to compensate for a controlled lifestyle. Everything is fine in moderation. I learnt all of this with Joe.

I hope that you have enjoyed this book. Through it all the spirit of Joe lingers. I have shed many tears, tears of joy for his life and the time that we were lucky enough to share. I hope that it has given you something, whether it be the strength to fight cancer in a different way or to make lifestyle changes to help you to keep your body as healthy as possible to fight the fights that it may have to face. Thank you for reading our story. May you have a long, healthy and happy life.

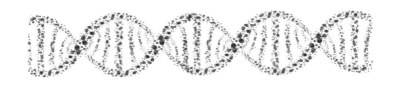

14 — Glossary

Abiraterone (Zytiga) — this is a newly approved hormone therapy which works to reduce androgens and is especially effective on metastatic prostate cancer which has not responded to chemotherapy which contains docetaxel (Taxotere). It is administered in tablet form and is usually administered with the anti–inflammatory drug prednisone which helps with some of the side–effects. It blocks an enzyme called cytochrome P17 and without this the body cannot make androgens i.e. cannot make testosterone and hence the cancer cells are not fed by this method.

Alprostadil — causes blood vessels to expand, increasing blood flow through the body. When injected into the penis it can facilitate an erection to enable sexual intercourse to take place. It can be used in conjunction with viagra.

Amygdalin (Laetrile) — is a plant substance found naturally in raw nuts and the pips of many fruits, particularly apricot pips, and is meant to reduce cancer's resistance to treatment and releases cyanide to kill cancer cells directly. This drug is not FDA approved and its claims are unsubstantiated by any published reports.

Androgens — these are hormones which control the development of the male characteristics. However, they are also present in females. The main androgens are testosterone and dihydrotestosterone. Androgens stimulate prostate cancer cells to grow. Certain hormone therapies are used in the fight against cancer by attempting to reduce the androgens which can reach the prostate gland.

Angiogenesis — is the growth of new blood vessels from pre-existent blood vessels which the cancer uses to obtain nutrients. They are created by proteins which promote this growth such as VEGF (vascular endothelial growth factor). VEGFs normal function is to create new blood vessels during embryonic development, to create new blood vessels following injury or to bypass blocked vessels.

Antioxidant — inhibits the oxidation of other cells and protects cells from free radicals by interacting with them, stabilizing them and eliminating them, thereby preventing cellular damage.

Apoptosis — programmed cell death. Cells within the body routinely die off and new cells form — this is the process which controls the balance between new and dying cells. It can also send signals for a damaged or infected cell to die.

Bevacizumab (Avastin) — this is an anti-body which inhibits VEGF (described in body of text). It is administered through an intravenous drip. It is often used in conjunction which docetaxel (Taxotere) chemotherapy. It is FDA approved for breast cancer and stage three clinical trials are underway for prostate cancer.

Bicalutamide (Casodex) — this is a hormone therapy. Cancer cells have receptors which testosterone attaches to and then the cancer cells can grow. Bicalutamide prevents the testosterone from attaching. It is administered in tablet form.

Biological therapy — uses the body's own immune system to fight the cancer. It uses biological response modifiers (which are grown in a laboratory) to 'talk to' the immune system and use it to stop the cancer growing, make cancer cells more recognisable so that they can be killed by the immune system, make immune system cells stronger and prevent cancer cells from spreading further afield in the body.

Bisphosphonates — zoledronic acid (Zometa) is an example of a bisphosphonate. In normal bones, two types of cells work together, one type (osteoclasts) destroying old bone and the other (osteoblasts) building new bone. This is a balancing act which is very tightly controlled within the body. However, some cancers can mean that the cells which destroy the bone work harder causing bone to become thin and weakened. Bisphosphonates target the areas where this imbalance is occurring and the osteoclasts absorb the bisphosphonates and slow down their activity. Bisphosphonates can slow down the spread of cancer in the bones and they reduce the risk of fracture. However, with long term use (over a year) a side-effect can be osteonecrosis of the jaw.

Bortezomib (Velcade) — is a proteasomes inhibitor. Proteasomes break down proteins and play an important part in cell function and growth. Interfering with how the proteasomes work can cause the cancer cells to die. It is administered by a subcutaneous injection or through an intravenous drip.

Brachytherapy — this is internal radiotherapy. For low dose radiation small radioactive seeds (between eighty and one hundred and twenty) are placed in the prostate gland. These give a localised dose of radiotherapy for a few months and then the radiation in the seeds runs out. For high dose radiation a tube is passed up the rectum (under general anaesthetic) and a high dose of radiotherapy is given directly into the prostate gland. This treatment is usually accompanied by external radiotherapy. Both of these methods provide localised radiotherapy and can only be used if the prostate cancer is early stage.

Carboplatin — this is a chemotherapy drug which is used in conjunction with docetaxel (Taxotere) in patients who have not responded to docetaxel (Taxotere) chemotherapy alone. It is administered through an intravenous drip.

Carcinogen — any substance which is directly involved in causing cancer

Chelation therapy — this involves the injection of a chemical into the patient's bloodstream which clings to the excess metals and plaque therein and cleans them out.

Chlorambucil (Leukeran) — this is a type of chemotherapy drug known as an alkylating agent. It is administered in tablet form. An alkylating agent sticks to the cancer cell's DNA and prevents it from replicating and hence helps to prevent the growth of the cancer.

Cores — the amount of cancer in prostate needle core tissue gives a good indication of the severity of the cancer and how best to manage it. Samples are taken using a core biopsy needle which has a slightly larger hole in the middle than a normal needle so that wider samples can be taken. The number of core samples which have a positive show of cancer provide an indication of the severity of the prognosis.

CTC — circulating tumour cells which are in the bloodstream and can lead to additional tumours elsewhere in the body. CTCs are the cells which escape from the primary tumour and are circulating in the blood stream. They can eventually settle down at a secondary site and cause metastasis.

Degarelix (Firmagon) — blocks the production of the luteinising hormone by the pituitary gland and hence lowers the level of testosterone in the blood and, since prostate cancer usually needs testosterone to grow, this is beneficial. It is administered as a subcutaneous injection. See hormone therapy treatment.

Dexamethasone — this is a steroid. Steroids are sometimes used when the prostate cancer is not responding to hormone therapy treatment and can be used alongside chemotherapy. It is also used for patients undergoing chemotherapy to counteract some of the side–effects, mainly inflammation as a reaction to the toxic drug. It is administered either in tablet form or as an injection.

Diethylstilbestrol (Stilboestrol) — this is a hormone therapy drug. It works by making the body think that it has too many male sex hormones and so the body stops producing them. It is administered in tablet form.

DNA — most of the work in our bodies is done by nutrients and proteins, but the DNA is the instruction manual telling them what to do. Half of your DNA is from your mother and the other half from your father — details such as the colour of your eyes, the shape of your nose. So this map of who you are is created to say how you should be created within the womb and how you should develop. It is like a computer programme so doesn't do anything itself but determines what everything else within your body does.

Docetaxel (Taxotere) — a liquid chemotherapy drug. It works by preventing the cancer cells from dividing into two i.e. multiplying and so slows the growth of the cancer. It is administered through an intravenous drip.

Electrolytes — these are minerals (such as calcium, magnesium, sodium) in your blood and other bodily fluids which carry an electric charge around your body. If the electric voltage is not correct then the signals which are passed between cells cannot be passed quickly enough and vital functions can break down. Electrolytes are quickly replaced by drinking fluids, but are also replaced by the foods which we eat.

Flare — a flare is a drug–induced reaction by the body to treatments being administered. Flares should be heeded as they can lead to serious complications if not dealt with.

Flutamide — see hormone therapy treatment

Free Radical — electrons in atoms are usually paired. A free radical is an atom which has unpaired electrons. They are therefore very reactive (as they look to find electrons to pair with) and can cause damage to surrounding molecules. A large number of free radicals can be an indication of cancer and can lead to cancer as they harm the DNA which can result in cell mutation.

Gamma knife treatment — a form of radiotherapy which delivers a high dose of radiation directly onto the affected area without damaging any surrounding tissue and without any incisions. It is not actually a knife but a specialised treatment system.

Gleason score — the Gleason score is a grading system used by pathologists to indicate how aggressive the cancer is. A biopsy sample is placed under a microscope and the pathologist assesses where the cancer is most prominent (the primary area) and where it is next most prominent (the secondary area). To each of these areas he will assign a number between 1 and 5 with 5 being the most advanced stage of cancer. So a Gleason score of 7 can be obtained, for example, by 3+4 or 4+3. The second of these two results is worse as it indicates that the cancer is more advanced in the primary area.

So it is always best to get the two numbers together rather than just the aggregate to be sure of the true situation. The higher the Gleason score the more aggressive is the cancer. Scores of two to four indicate a cancer which is low on the aggression scale, scores of five and six are mildly aggressive. A score of seven indicates that the cancer is moderately aggressive. Scores between eight and ten mean that the cancer is very aggressive.

Goserelin (Zoladex) — is a hormone therapy and is used for many forms of cancer including prostate cancer. It is administered as a subcutaneous injection. Production of testosterone is stimulated by a hormone called a luteinising hormone. A luteinising hormone blocker (see hormone replacement therapy), goserelin stops the production of this luteinising hormone and therefore works well in conjunction with other hormone therapies which prevent the production of testosterone. It is also given to treat prostate cancer which has spread to the area surrounding the prostate gland (locally advanced).

Hormone therapy treatment — prostate cancer depends on testosterone to grow. Hormone therapy treatment attempts to reduce the amount of testosterone being produced. It is not usually needed for early stage prostate cancer and is usually employed where the cancer has spread beyond the prostate gland itself, the PSA level at diagnosis was very high and/or the Gleason score is high. The treatment is given for periods of anything between three months and a number of years depending upon the patient's response, as the cancer can simply stop responding to the hormone therapy treatment after a period of time i.e. it becomes immune to it. There are four main types of drug which are used:

Abiraterone (Zytiga) — described above

Luteinising hormone (LH) blocker — goserelin (Zoladex) is one example. The pituitary gland in the brain releases a hormone which tells the testes to make testosterone. This treatment stops the pituitary gland from making the hormone.

Gonadotropin releasing hormone (GnRH) blocker — Degarelix (Firmagon) is an example. This treatment stops the message which the hormone released by the pituitary gland sends to the testes to make testosterone.

Anti-androgens — flutamide and bicalutamide are examples. This treatment starves the cancer cells of testosterone which prevents them from growing and eventually this causes the tumour to shrink.

Lapatinib (Tyverb) — a tyrosine kinase inhibitor which targets HER2. It works by blocking the signals within the cancer cells which tell them to divide which causes the cells to die. As with Bevacizumab (Avastin), it is used in breast cancer treatment and not currently used in orthodox prostate cancer treatment. It is administered in tablet form.

Lesion — there are many forms of lesion but they are basically a localised, abnormal change in the body, either in bone, tissue or organ. In the case of X–ray or MRI imaging it describes scarring to the bone which can be caused by cancer or other diseases such as multiple sclerosis, or it can indeed be simply due to the wear and tear of ageing. The radiographer can assess which type of lesion is being seen on the scans by using their training.

Lomustine — this is a type of chemotherapy drug known as an alkylating agent. An alkylating agent sticks to the cancer cell's DNA and prevents it from replicating. It is administered in tablet form.

Metastasis/Metastatic/Metastasised — the spread of cancer from its original site.

Mastitis — is the inflammation of the mammary gland and udder tissue of dairy cattle. It usually occurs as an immune response to bacterial invasion of the teat canal by bacteria, and can occur as a result of chemical, mechanical, or thermal injury to a cow's udder.

PCA3 — this is a new test based on DNA technology which provides a more efficient means of detecting prostate cancer than the standard PSA test. This urine test can help to avoid the need for unnecessary prostate biopsies.

PET Scan — Positron Emission Tomography — this type of scan can show how body tissues are working as well as what they are. These scans are not readily available in the UK as they are expensive. Following treatment for cancer, a CT scan may show that there are still some signs of cancer remaining. However, this may not be live cancer and may just be leftover dead tissue. A PET scan will show whether the tissue is still active cancer whereas a CT scan will not.

Phytochemicals — these are plant chemicals which have protective or disease–preventing properties. The body doesn't need them to survive. There are many different types of phytochemicals which have varying properties such as antioxidant (fruit, vegetables), enzyme stimulator (cabbage, soya, beans), interferer of DNA replication preventing the division of cancer cells (beans, hot peppers) and anti–bacterial properties (allicin from garlic).

Prostate — the prostate is part of the male reproductive system and is situated just below the bladder. It produces fluid which protects sperm. Prostate cancer occurs when some cells within the prostate reproduce too rapidly and create a swelling or tumour. The cancer is controllable if discovered at this stage. The problem occurs when these cells break free and attack other areas of the body like the lymph nodes and bones.

Prostatectomy — the removal of the prostate gland by surgery

Prostatitis — this is inflammation of the prostate and surrounding area. Whereas prostate cancer can be life–threatening, prostatitis is benign (not life–threatening). It is caused by swelling of the prostate and can cause discomfort in the pelvis. It is difficult to differentiate between prostatitis and prostate cancer simply from a rectal examination.

PSA — Prostate–Specific Antigen — is a substance produced by the prostate gland. A blood test is performed to assess whether levels are elevated which could indicate prostate cancer, but it could also indicate prostatitis or enlarged prostate. Also, men with cancer may not show elevated PSA levels. Further tests should be performed in conjunction with this test. A level of below four has generally been accepted as normal. However, PSA levels in younger men are lower so the ceiling for results should be lowered in such cases.

Rilutek — this is a promising drug in hard to treat cancers (triple negative breast, melanoma). It has been used in combination with other agents in uncontrollable cancer. In general, it has two functions — the first is to block the release of substances needed for the proliferation of cancer cells and, with such action, trigger apoptosis of cancer cells, the second is to regulate the glutamate signal. Glutamine is in abundance in food and blocking absorption through glutamate receptor signalling prevents absorption of glutamate and other unwanted amino acids by rapidly dividing cancer cells.

Sorafenib (Nexavar) — a tyrosine kinase inhibitor. It is administered in tablet form. It works by blocking the signals within the cancer cells which tell them to divide which causes the cells to die. After a time, hormone therapy may no longer be effective against cancer cell division. The cancer evolves and learns how to use different methods to grow. It can use proteins to help the cells divide and survive. By blocking the tyrosine kinase enzymes, which activate the proteins, it can deny the cells a means of growth. This drug is also an angiogenesis inhibitor.

Teriparatide (Forteo) — a bone formation agent used to treat osteoporosis and prevent bone loss. It is administered as an injection.

Tumour — this is a lump or growth of tissue which consists of abnormal cells. Tumours are divided into two types — malignant (which are potentially life-threatening) and benign (not life-threatening).

Viagra — a medication used to treat erectile dysfunction and to help gain and sustain an erection. It is often used following the prostatectomy to help to gain an erection and can sometimes be used in conjunction with a penile injection of alprostadil.

Vorinostat — is a type of anti-cancer drug known as a histone deacetylase (HDAC) inhibitor. Cancer cells sometimes have too many of these enzymes which stop the cells from making proteins needed to keep them from growing and dividing too fast.

Zoledronic Acid (Zometa) — see bisphosphonates. It is administered through an intravenous drip.

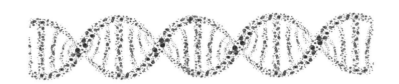

15 — Appendix

Appendix 1 – Extract by Dr Seeger

The Arrest of Cancer

In order to arrest cancer you need to know how cancer cells work and their defence mechanisms against our immune system and whatever treatment we apply to combat them. There are about two hundred different forms of cancer in the human body known and there is one thing which they all have in common — anaerobic cell metabolism. End product of anaerobic cell metabolism is lactic acid.

To this very day we do not know the mechanism by which the oxygen molecule leaves the blood vessel and how they get transported to cells in exchange for the waste product CO_2 at cellular level. We know how it works in the lung but this model cannot be applied to other tissues. Austrian Professor Alfred Pischinger has described a model of extra–cellular space (now known as 'Pischinger space') that connects the whole body. This is where it's all happening. All things which cells need to function properly, such as oxygen, nutrients, vitamins and trace elements must be transported through the extra–cellular space between blood vessels and cells in exchange for waste products from the cell that are somehow moved to and into the blood vessel.

As mentioned above, cancer cells have an anaerobic cell metabolism so there is a big build–up of lactic acid around a cancerous tumour. Lactic acid is also produced when we overwork our muscles into the anaerobic zone. Most of us know the resulting muscle soreness but we also know it will subside with rest. The difference with cancer cells is that there is no rest. Lactic acid is produced 24/7 and the normal physiological mechanisms to neutralise it soon fail and a lactic acid shield is mounted around the tumour. This lactic acid shield prevents our own self–defence against cancer cells, the killer T–Cell Lymphocytes, from penetrating cancer cells by releasing perforin to destroy it. At the same time, it prevents any useful adjuvants that show in vitro anti–cancer properties to do the same thing.

Once I understood how cancer cells shield themselves against attacks it was easy to plan a counter attack. Most alternative cancer treatments that claim success these days involve alkaline diets and alkaline drinks. Let's face it, the most boring foods and most nauseating drinks on this planet are alkaline. So it takes a super human effort to sustain it and only the very few who have done it can claim success. Make no mistake, I am not saying I have a treatment where people can eat and drink whatever they like but they can be a bit more relaxed about it. It's all about quality of life. I don't want to live to one hundred if I'm only allowed wheatgrass juice, vegetable juices, green tea, raw veggies and coffee enemas.

The pH of the human blood is kept by physiological mechanisms between 7.35 and 7.45. If the pH drops below 7.32 for a prolonged period of time the person will die. Even in cancer patients with this massive acid build–up the human body will try to keep this blood pH. This comes at an enormous cost to other organs. Alkaline minerals like calcium, magnesium, manganese or alkaline trace elements like selenium etc. are used up to counteract the acid onslaught. Taking all of this into account, it makes sense to administer intravenous alkaline infusions to cancer patients. This is not something I have invented but is used frequently in medical conditions where certain events, e.g. metabolic acidosis, severe renal disease, hyperglycaemic coma and so on lead to an extra–cellular acid shift. Alkaline infusions can be bought ready–made by pharmaceutical companies like Pfizer's 8.4% Sodium Bicarbonate Solution. The skill is in which fashion to administer it to cancer patients. From the above it also makes sense to add things like alkaline minerals, essential trace elements and other things to the solution. How to dilute it in normal saline is also important, along with how fast to infuse it and at what temperature. It is also important to alternate these infusions with Vitamin C (plus other ingredients) infusions to eliminate waste products caused by the breakdown of the acid shield.

As you can tell, I am not giving away all of my knowledge on how to arrest cancer, but I have shown several times that it works. The problem is that this treatment is not covered by any health fund.

People feel better in a short period of time and after a couple of months they are so well that they think they can now just do it on their own with some vegetable juices and a few supplements. It takes on average seven years for cancer to be diagnosed — so whoever thinks I can cure it in two months please do not contact me!

Well, that's my story, and that's why I have gone back to my old trade, Orthopaedic Surgery.

Hilbert Seeger, M.D. Ph.D.
drseeger@gmail.com
Input from Dr Seeger: Dr Hilbert Seegers Dark Field Microscopy Live Blood Analysis Training Course
www.livebloodtraining.com/

The prime cause and prevention of cancer
Dr. Otto Warburg
Lecture delivered to Nobel Laureates on June 30, 1966 at Lindau, Lake Constance, Germany

…….. Cancer, above all other diseases, has countless secondary causes. Almost anything can cause cancer. But, even for cancer, there is only one prime cause. The prime cause of cancer is the replacement of the respiration of oxygen (oxidation of sugar) in normal body cells by fermentation of sugar.

All normal body cells meet their energy needs by respiration of oxygen, whereas cancer cells meet their energy needs in great part by fermentation. All normal body cells are thus obligate aerobes, whereas all cancer cells are partial anaerobes. ………………

……….. All carcinogens impair respiration directly or indirectly by deranging capillary circulation, a statement that is proven by the fact that no cancer cell exists without exhibiting impaired respiration. Of course, respiration cannot be repaired if it is impaired at the same time by a carcinogen. …………………..

Dr. Seeger's notes:

This statement has never been scientifically challenged, which means it is generally accepted that mitochondria of cancer cells have lost ability to use oxygen for energy and need to switch to anaerobic cell metabolism. The end product of this is lactic acid. So there is a massive build–up of lactic acid around a tumour, which forms a protective shield around it making it hard for cancer destructive agents to reach it. Generally, therefore, cancer patients become very acidic over time. This is why alkaline foods and drinks are always recommended in natural therapies. So far it doesn't seem to have bearing in conventional cancer treatment.

For a most effective treatment of cancer patients I have taken these facts into account and came up with intravenous bicarbonate infusions with many other ingredients in it alternating with vitamin C infusions. Why this is so effective in arresting cancer is described in my statement: 'Arresting cancer or call it a cure — if you can afford it'.

Input from Dr Seeger: Dr Hilbert Seegers Dark Field Microscopy Live Blood Analysis Training Course
www.livebloodtraining.com/

Acid Stress

Almost every biological process in a human body depends on the acid–base balance in the extra–cellular fluids. Modern western diets lead to chronic, low–grade metabolic acidosis. With advancing age, the severity of diet–dependent acidosis increases independently of diet because of declining kidney function.

In illness, the shifts in the acid–base metabolism become even more relevant.

The typical Western diet is usually a net producer of non–carbonic acids not only because of its large content of acid–generating animal proteins, but also because of large amounts of cereal grain products and relatively lower amounts of bicarbonate–generating plant foods. Although the pre–modern diet contained considerable amounts of meat, it was a net producer of bicarbonate because it also contained large amounts of fruit and vegetables that generated substantial amounts of bicarbonate via metabolism. Accordingly, humans evolved to excrete large loads of bicarbonate and potassium, not the large net acid loads chronically generated by the current Western dietary patterns.

The renal acidification process in humans does not completely excrete the modern acid load. The unexcreted acid does not titrate plasma bicarbonate to ever lower concentrations, but rather to sustain concentrations only slightly lower than those that otherwise occur. This is because the unexcreted hydrogen ion not only exchanges with bone sodium and potassium, but also titrates and is neutralized by basic salts of bone. Although preventing the occurrence of frank metabolic acidosis, the acid titration of calcium containing carbonates and hydroxyapatite mobilizes bone calcium and over time dissolves bone matrix. The buffering by bone of diet-derived acid may be regarded as a biological trade-off.

At the cost of bone demineralization, arterial pH and plasma bicarbonate concentration are only modestly reduced by an acidogenic diet, such as the Western-type diet, and not to values below their 'normal' range. These normal reduced values, however, reflect a state of low-grade metabolic acidosis.

In plain English, you do not have to suffer from metabolic acidosis and be treated in Intensive Care to feel the ill health effects of latent acidosis/systemic hyperacidity or, as I call it, 'Acid Stress', and Acid Stress makes you sick!

The Clinical Picture of Acid Stress

The pH of different tissues and body fluids varies, for example, normal pH of the skin is about 5.5, of the vagina about 2 and in the stomach around 1.5–3. Most important is the pH of the blood, because it must be kept constant for the body to function properly. If this pH drops below 7.28 the blood cells begin to degenerate.

The pH of the human blood plasma is normally between 7.37 and 7.43. The red blood cell pH, which is hard to measure, is around 7.29. The blood has several buffer systems, which keep the acid-base household in balance and the pH within this range. With the uptake of acid forming foodstuff like wheat, meat, cheese, coffee, sugar etc., bases are needed to neutralize these acids. Alkaline minerals (mainly calcium and magnesium) are drawn from tissues. As a result of constant over-supply of acid-forming foods, lots of alkaline minerals will be drawn from the tissues, leaving them in an acidic state. It comes as no surprise that most gout attacks, which is a dump of excess uric acid, occur over the Christmas holidays.

The overall metabolism of human beings is slightly acidic because of the endogenous (produced or grown from within) production of acids. The blood plasma pH on the other hand is slightly alkaline. To maintain this slightly alkaline pH, acid must be constantly excreted in the urine. Therefore, the average pH of the urine is markedly lower.

Some time following food intake, excess bicarbonate produced by the pancreas is absorbed in the small intestine. The pancreas produces less sacharases (enzymes needed to digest sugar) at night. Therefore, the sugar in fruit consumed in the evening cannot be readily absorbed but must be glycolised and fermented by intestinal bacteria.

Intestinal fermentation plays a major part in the endogenous formation of acids. It results from excessive sugar intake and leads to the formation of lactic acid.

The majority of exogenous oversupply of acids, however, is due to excessive intake of meat (animal protein). Some problems are caused by phosphate, which binds with alkaline minerals, others by the lack of alkaline foods and alkaline minerals in the diet.

Mechanisms of Acid Excretion

To guarantee a proper acid–base balance, the body must excrete the acids that are formed by your metabolism. The kidneys usually do this. At night sour urine is excreted and during the day it should be around the neutral range. If there is an increased acid production or too much intake of acid–forming foods, the urine will be constantly in a sour range and the normal physiological alkaline peaks of the urine cease.

Kidneys / Uro-genital System

Constant sour urine promotes irritation of the mucosa, chronic cystitis and genital infections as well as genital mycosis, and in males a latent chronic irritation of the prostate. All these ailments therefore respond very well to a consequent alkalizing therapy. Particularly elderly female patients with chronic cystitis can be cured of this within about one year and always without antibiotics.

If the kidneys can't cope with the excretion of all that acid — this can be demonstrated by measuring the urine pH, which is then always in an acidic range — other excretory organs must help to eliminate acid. This leads to pH changes of sweat, stools, bronchials and other excretory systems.

Stomach

The stomach reacts to systemic hyperacidity with hydrogen chloride excretion even during digestion-free periods. This undue release of hydrogen chloride leads to gastritis and later to stomach and duodenal ulcers. Increased excretion of acid in the stomach is one way for the body to eliminate sour substances and should never be suppressed with H2-blockers because this acid remains in the body and leads to an acidosis of the tissues and an overload of the buffer mechanisms of the blood. Instead the hyperacidity of the stomach should be treated long-term with sodium bicarbonate preparations and essential trace elements and stimulation of the physiological bicarbonate production of the pancreas. It is also important to eliminate animal proteins as much as possible from the diet because these proteins stimulate hydrogen chloride and pepsin excretion of the stomach additionally.

Skin

The skin reacts to systemic hyperacidity with the production of sour sweat. There is also an increased excretion of proteins in the sweat and this leads to irritations of the skin, changes of the pH of the skin and toxic reactions of the skin. Eczema, allergic skin reactions and dermatitis are often consequences of systemic hyperacidity. Patients with this sort of complaint should therefore always be treated with an alkalizing therapy combined with a treatment of the intestinal mucosa.

Airways

The mucosa of the rhino-bronchial system can also be part of the mechanism of acid excretion in systemic hyperacidity. This establishes itself in an increase in bronchial secretion and viscous sinual mucous with a tendency to recurrent bronchitis and sinusitis. The viscosity of the mucous depends on its acid content. Consequences are a hyperactive bronchial system and asthmatic tendencies.

Intestines

The intestines are the biggest mucosal organ of the body and also the biggest excretory organ. The secretion of the small intestine amounts to approximately twenty litres per day. The larger part of this is usually reabsorbed in the ileum and the colon. The acid content of the small intestine is normally in a pH range of 6.0–6.8. This shows that a lot of acid excretion takes place in the small intestine. This acid should ideally be neutralized by the food mash. Therefore, it is important to have a lot of alkaline minerals and non–absorbable alkaline fibres in the diet. These neutralize acid by forming phytates and other fibre complexes, which are than excreted with the stools. Otherwise some of the acid is reabsorbed into the body and the faeces in the colon is very acidic. This may lead to colitis or an irritable colon. Therefore, the diet of a patient suffering from colitis or irritable colon should always be changed to an alkaline fibre–rich and animal protein free diet. This change in diet must be done slowly to avoid any adverse reactions of the already hypersensitive intestines.

Food allergies — mostly against dairy products — should also be taken into consideration and treated. Every food allergy causes a villous atrophy and again leads to an increased reabsorption of acids.

Joints, Muscles & Bones

Every joint has a capsule around it. The inner lining of the capsule, the synovial membrane, produces joint grease (synovial). Yet another mechanism of a body suffering from systemic hyperacidity is the discharge of acidic substances through the synovial membranes. If the sour substance produced is uric acid it expresses itself as gout. But it can also be other forms of acid. This always causes an inflammatory reaction. Examinations of aspirated fluid from these joints by dark field microscopy show highly developed endobiontic structures and a rapid formation of spicules as well as various crystalline structures, an indication of hyperacidity of the milieu.

Osteoporosis is not just a disturbance of the bone metabolism but a problem of systemic hyperacidity as well. Overseas studies show that osteoporosis can be treated successfully with diet, an alkalizing therapy plus medication to improve the bone metabolism.

Consequences of Systemic Hyperacidity

Constant systemic hyperacidity leads to de–calcification of bones and calcifications in muscles, connective tissues, joint capsules and blood vessels (arteriosclerosis).

The withdrawal of cationic trace elements selenium, zinc, magnesium, calcium, manganese — the ones that are used up to bind oversupplies of acids and proteins — leads to osteoporosis, degeneration of cartilage and a lack of trace elements. As a result, the binding sites that are usually occupied by these trace elements can become occupied by toxic trace elements or heavy metals. Therefore, mercury, aluminium and lead poisoning can establish itself much more severely if systemic hyperacidity is present. Therefore, heavy metal poisoning must always be treated with an alkalizing therapy as well.

Reference: *Dr Hilbert Seeger's Dark Field Microscopy Live Blood Analysis Training Course*
Author:Hilbert Seeger, MD, PhD
E-mail: drseeger@gmail.com

Appendix 2 — Bibliography from Dr Hilu

Hyperthermia Bibliography:

Back up information:

ICHO 2008 (International Congress On Hyperthermic Oncology)
ESHO 2009 (European Society for Hyperthermic Oncology)
ESHO 2010 (European Society for Hyperthermic Oncology)
STM 2010 (Society for Thermal Medicine)
www.vci.org
www.esho.infowww.thermaltherapy.org
www.jstage.jst.go.jp/browse/thermalmed
www.rsny.org

- 1. Kampinga HH, Konings AWT: Inhibition of repair of X-ray induced DNA damage by heat: the role of hyperthermic inhibition of DNA polymerase activity. Rad Res, 112: 86-98, 1987.

- 2. Kampinga HH, Dynlacht JR, Dikomey E: Mechanism of radiosensitization (43 °C) as derived from studies with DNA repair defective mutant cell lines. Int J Hyperthermia, 20: 131-139, 2004.

- 3. Kampinga HH: Cell biological effects of hyperthermia alone or combined with radiation or drugs: A short introduction to newcomers in the field. Int J Hyperthermia, 22: 191-196, 2006.

- 4. Borys N: Phase I/II study evaluating the xtrace tolerated dose, pharmacokinetics, safety, and efficacy of approved hyperthermia and lyso-thermosensitive liposomal doxorubicin in patients with breast xtrac recurrence at the chest wall. ASCO abstracts book, 2010.

- 5. Vaupel P, Otte J, Manz R: Changes in tumor oxygenation after localized microwave heating. Prog Clin Biol Res, 107: 65-74, 1982.

- 6. Bicher HI, Mitagvaria NP, Bruley DF: Changes in tumor tissue oxygenation during microwave hyperthermia: clinical relevance. Adv Exp Med Biol, 180: 901-905, 1984.

- 7. Wahl ML, Bobyock SB, Leeper DB, Owen CS: Effects of 42 degrees C hyperthermia on xtracelular pH in xtrace carcinoma cells during acute or chronic exposure to low xtracelular pH. Int J Radiat Oncol Biol Phys, 39: 205-212, 1997.

- 8. Nakano H, Kurihara K, Okamoto M, Toné S, Shinohara K: Heat-induced apoptosis and p53 in cultured mammalian cells. Int J Radiat Oncol Biol Phys, 71: 519-529, 1997.

- 9. Coss RA, Sedar AW, Sistrun SS, Storck CW, Wang PH, Wachsberger PR: Hsp27 protects the cytoskeleton and nucleus from the effects of 42 degrees C at pH 6.7 in CHO cells adapted to growth at pH 6.7. Int J Hyperthermia, 18: 216-232, 2002.

- 10. Dayanc BE, Beachy SH, Ostberg JR, Repasky EA: Dissecting the role of hyperthermia in natural killer cell mediated anti-tumor responses. Int J Hyperthermia, 24: 41-56, 2008.

- 11. Hetzel FW, Mattiello J: Interactions of hyperthermia with other modalities. In: Medical physics monograph n° 16. Biological, physical and clinical aspects of hyperthermia. Paliwal BR, Hetzel FW and Dewhirst MW (Eds), pp 30-56, Am Inst Phys, 1987.

- 12. Manning MR, Cetas TC, Miller RC, Oleson JR, Connor WG, Gerner EW: Clinical hyperthermia: results of a phase I trial employing hyperthermia alone or in combination with external beam or interstitial radiotherapy. Cancer, 49: 205-216, 1982.

- 13. Dunlop PRC, Hand JW, Dickinson RJ, Field SB: An assessment of local hyperthermia in clinical practise. Int J Hyperthermia, 2: 39-50, 1986.

- 14. Gabriele P, Orecchia R, Ragona R, Tseroni V, Sannazzari GL: Hyperthermia alone in the treatment of recurrence of malignant tumors. Cancer, 66: 2191-2195, 1990.

Formula DEG Bibliography

- 1.Leung A, Foster S. Encyclopedia of Common Natural Ingredients Used in Food, Drugs and Cosmetics, 2d ed. New York: John Wiley & Sons, 1996, 113-4.

- 2.Weiss RF. Herbal Medicine. Gothenburg, Sweden: Ab Arcanum, 1988, 344.

- 3.Della Loggia R, Tubaro A, Sosa S, et al. The role of triterpenoids in the topical anti-inflammatory activity of Calendula officinalis flowers. Planta Med 1994;60:516-20.

- 4.Bogdanova NS, Nikolaeva IS, Shcherbakova LI, et al. Study of antiviral properties of Calendula officinalis.Farmskolto Ksikol 1970;33:349-55 [in Russian].

- 5.De Tommasi N, Conti C, Stein ML, et al. Structure and in vitro activity of triterpenoid saponins form Calendulaarvensis. Plants Med 1991;57:250-3.

- 6.Wichtl M. Herbal Drugs and Phytopharmaceuticals. Boca Raton, FL: CRC Press, 1994, 118-200

Appendix 3 — Poly MVA

Poly-MVA is a promising new dietary supplement that may assist in boosting immune response, and healing damaged cells. It is a uniquely formulated nutritional supplement containing a proprietary blend of Palladium and alpha–lipoic acid (which we refer to as LAPd), Vitamins B1, B2 and B12, formylmethionine, acetyl cystiene, and trace amounts of molybdinum, rhodium, and ruthenium. It is designed to provide energy for compromised body systems by changing the electrical potential of human cells, increasing the charge density of DNA within the cell.

Poly-MVA is a new, non–toxic, powerful antioxidant dietary supplement. While definitive studies on its effect in human nutrition and health are under way, early studies and anecdotal information indicate that the active ingredients in Poly-MVA may be beneficial in protecting cell DNA and RNA, assisting the body in producing energy, and providing support to the liver in removing harmful substances from the body.

Some studies indicate that ingredients of Poly-MVA can assist in preventing cell damage, and removing heavy metals from the bloodstream. As a powerful antioxidant, it can help to neutralise the free radicals within the body that are thought to influence the ageing process and convert them into energy. Other ingredients are involved in DNA synthesis, production of the myelin sheath that protects nerves, red blood cell production and playing an important role in immune and nerve function.

What makes Poly-MVA unique is the special, proprietary manufacturing process by which lipoic acid is bonded to Palladium (LAPd). No other company produces any product similar to Poly-MVA because of the patented preparation and bonding process through which LAPd is manufactured. The proprietary formulation of LAPd with other vitamins, minerals, and amino acids provides considerable nutritional support, helping to enable optimum functioning of essential body systems.

Poly-MVA can provide the following nutritional support to the body:

- Helps the body to produce energy
- Supports the liver in removing harmful substances from the body

- Assists in preventing cell damage
- Assists the body in removing heavy metals from the bloodstream
- Powerful antioxidant and detoxificant
- Prevents B-12 deficiency related mental disturbances in the elderly
- Supports nerve and neurotransmitter function
- Enhances white blood cell function
- Supports pH balance, helping to maintain oxygenation of cells and tissues

Although not all scientific studies have been completed, a significant number of articles in peer–reviewed scientific and medical journals discuss the possible biochemical significance of LAPd in supporting various biological functions within animals and humans. Additionally, some studies have already been planned or are currently underway to further evaluate the value and effectiveness of LAPd in human nutrition.

Appendix 4 — Cellfood

Cellfood is the world's number one selling oxygen and nutrient supplement. For more than forty years, NuScience Corporation has manufactured Everett Storey's original Cellfood formula containing seventy–eight minerals, thirty–four enzymes, and seventeen amino acids. Cellfood utilises a proprietary water–splitting technology that provides a powerful stream of bio–available oxygen plus one hundred and twenty–nine nutrients directly to the cells.

Free radicals are atoms (or groups of atoms) that are missing an electron. These highly reactive molecules become even more dangerous in the human body when they react with and damage other important cellular components like DNA. Antioxidants are directly responsible for the prevention of cellular damage by neutralising and eliminating free radicals. In a recent study, Cellfood was shown to decrease excess free radical activity by up to 27%. Cellfood's colloidal and ionic formula has a negative charge (as measure by Zeta potential testing). This negatively charged solution (like blood and lymph) allows for the rapid absorption and assimilation of nutrients. This process enables the body to more efficiently eliminate toxins and balance PH.

In addition to the numerous general health benefits, Cellfood has now become the supplement of choice for many professional athletes. In a study conducted at the University of Pretoria, Cellfood was shown to increase oxygen uptake (VO2 Max), increase ferretin (iron storage), and decrease lactic acid accumulation (muscular fatigue). Cellfood is made from the finest all–natural, plant–based organic substances. Cellfood contains no alcohol, glucose, yeast, or gluten. Cellfood does not contain any ingredients that are on the 'list of banned substances' for professional and amateur athletic competitions and associations. Cellfood is non–addictive, non–invasive, and completely non–toxic.'

Appendix 5 — Formula Immune

It is manufactured by RayRos.com. It contains 80% arabinogalactans and 20% non–acidifying vitamin C.

Arabinogalactans have been highly researched both as prebiotics, immune system boosters as well as anti–cancer supplements (there are more than 22,000 publications that back up such investigations) Here are some references:

- Adams MF, Ettling BV. Industrial Gums 2nd Edition; Academic Press 1973.

- Ghoneum, M., Ghonaim, M., Namatalla, G. et al.: Natural Killer cell activity in hepatocellular carcinoma and its relation to the etiology of the hemstone. Theoretical Basis for Process Improvement with Chemstone OAE Technology.

- 3Tsao D, Shi Z, Wong A, Kim YS. Effect of sodium butyrate on carcinoembryonic antigen production by human colonic adenocarcinoma cells in xtrace. Cancer Res 1983;43:1217-1222.

- Kelly GS. Larch arabinogalactan: Clinical relevance of a novel immune-enhancing polysaccharide. Alternative Med Rev 1994; 4(2):96-103.

- Hauer J, Anderer FA. Mechanism of stimulation of human natural killer cytotoxicity by arabinogalactan from Larix occidentalis. Cancer Immunol Immunother 1993;36:237-244.

- Hagmar B, Ryd W, Skomedal H. Arabinogalactan blockade of experimental metastases to liver by murine hepatoma. Invasion Metastasis 1991;11:348-355

- Beuth J, Ko HL, Schirrmacher V,et al. Inhibition of liver tumor cell colonization in two animal tumor models by lectin blocking with D-galactose or arabinogalactan. Clin Exp Metastasis 1988;6:115-120.

- Levine PH, Whiteside TL,Friberg D, et al. Dysfunction of natural killer cell activity in a family with chronic fatigue xtracel. Clin Immunol Immunopathol 1998;88:96-104.

Appendix 6 — Papimi Machine

The Papimi — NanoPulse Therapy system is a medical device producing electromagnetic pulses, invented by the Greek Professor Dr Panos Pappas. It restores the electric potential of the cells, which in turn regulates the chemical interchanges towards normality in instances of disequilibrium. As a consequence the biochemical cellular processes are normalised, eliminating the associated symptoms, thus curing the illness. In other words it brings back into balance the body's electro–magnetic field.

The Papimi — Nanopulse therapy system is a most effective pulsed electromagnetic field therapy device. In particular, it produces short–duration and high–intensity magnetic pulses that penetrate in the body's tissues and increase the cells' ability to absorb ions. As a result, the system has the unique characteristic of being effective for a wide variety of health problems.

In the following link you can find various documented studies: _www.papimi.com/CASESen.htm_

You can also watch several videos explaining the theory and presenting testimonies from all around the globe at the following links: _www.papimi.com/Videos.htm_

The system is fully approved as a medical device Class Iia and it can be used in any private or public hospital/clinic/practice, or for personal use. _www.papimi.com/APPROVALSen.html_

To sum up, the Papimi — Nanopulse Therapy System is an excellent equipment to assist any health professional who is practicing alternative and holistic methods.

Appendix 7 – Top Ten Food Additives to Avoid

- Artificial Sweeteners
  Aspartame (E951), more popularly known as NutraSweet and Equal, is often found in foods labelled 'diet' or 'sugar free'. Aspartame is believed to be carcinogenic and accounts for more reports of adverse reactions than all other foods and food additives combined. Aspartame is not your friend. Aspartame is a neurotoxin and carcinogen. Known to erode intelligence and affect short–term memory, the components of this toxic sweetener may lead to a wide variety of ailments including brain tumour, diseases like lymphoma, diabetes, multiple sclerosis, Parkinson's, Alzheimer's, fibromyalgia and chronic fatigue, emotional disorders like depression and anxiety attacks, dizziness, headaches, nausea, mental confusion, migraines and seizures.

  Acesulfame–K, a relatively new artificial sweetener found in baking goods, gum and xtrace, has not been thoroughly tested and has been linked to kidney tumours. It is found in: diet or sugar free sodas, diet coke, coke zero, jello (and over gelatins), desserts, sugar free gum, drink mixes, baking goods, table top sweeteners, cereal, breath mints, pudding, kook–aid, ice tea, chewable vitamins and toothpaste.

- High Fructose Corn Syrup
  High fructose corn syrup (HFCS) is a highly–refined artificial sweetener which has become the number one source of calories in America. It is found in almost all processed foods. HFCS packs on the pounds faster than any other ingredient, increases your LDL ('bad') cholesterol levels and contributes to the developments of diabetes and tissue damage, among other harmful effects. It is found in: most processed foods, breads, candy, flavoured yoghurts, salad dressings, canned vegetables and cereals.

- Monosodium Glutamate (MSG/E621)
  MSG is an amino acid used as a flavour enhancer in soups, salad dressings, chips, frozen entrees and many restaurant foods. MSG is known as an excitotoxin, a substance which overexcites cells to the point of damage or death. Studies

show that regular consumption of MSG may result in adverse side effects which include depression, disorientation, eye damage, fatigue, headaches and obesity. MSG affects the neurological pathways of the brain and disengages the 'I'm full' function which explains the effects of weight gain. It is found in: Chinese food (Chinese restaurant syndrome) many snacks, chips, cookies, seasonings, some tinned soups, frozen dinners and lunch meats.

- Trans Fat
  Trans fat is used to enhance and extend the shelf life of food products and is among the most dangerous substances that you can consume. Found in deep–fried fast foods and certain processed foods made with margarine or partially hydrogenated vegetable oils, trans fats are formed by a process called hydrogenation. Numerous studies show that trans fat increases LDL cholesterol levels while decreasing HDL ('good') cholesterol, increases the risk of heart attacks, heart disease and strokes, and contributes to increased inflammation, diabetes and other health problems. Oils and fat are now forbidden on the Danish market if they contain fatty acids exceeding two per cent, a move that effectively bans partially hydrogenated oils. It is found in: margarine, chips and crackers, baked goods and fast foods.

- Common Food Dyes
  Studies show that artificial colourings which are found in soda, fruit juices and salad dressings, may contribute to behavioural problems in children and lead to a significant reduction in IQ. Animal studies have linked other food colourings to cancer. Watch out for these: Blue #1 and Blue #2 (E133) was banned in Norway, Finland and France. It may cause chromosomal damage. They are found in: candy, cereal, soft drinks, sports drinks and pet foods. Red dye #3 (also Red #40) (E124) was banned in 1990 after eight years of debate from use in many foods and cosmetics. This dye continues to be on the market until supplies run out. It has been proven to cause thyroid cancer and chromosomal damage in laboratory animals, and may also interfere with brain-nerve transmission. They are found in: fruit cocktail, maraschino cherries, cherry pie mix, ice cream, candy,

bakery products and more! Yellow #6 (E110) and Yellow Tartrazine (E102) were banned in Norway and Sweden. They increase the number of kidney and adrenal gland tumours in laboratory animals and may cause chromosomal damage. They are found in: American cheese, macaroni and cheese, candy and carbonated beverages, lemonade and more.

- Sodium Sulphite (E221)
Preservative used in wine–making and other processed foods. According to the FDA, approximately one in one hundred people is sensitive to sulphites in food. The majority of these individuals are asthmatic, suggesting a link between asthma and sulphites. Individuals who are sulphite sensitive may experience headaches, breathing problems, and rashes. In severe cases, sulphites can actually cause death by closing down the airway altogether, leading to cardiac arrest. It is found in: wine and dried fruit.

- Sodium Nitrate/Sodium Nitrite
Sodium nitrate (or sodium nitrite) is used as a preservative, colouring and flavouring in bacon, ham, hot dogs, luncheon meats, corned beef, smoked fish and other processed meats. This ingredient, which sounds harmless, is actually highly carcinogenic once it enters the human digestive system. There, it forms a variety of nitrosamine compounds that enter the bloodstream and wreak havoc on a number of internal organs, the liver and pancreas in particular. Sodium nitrite is widely regarded as a toxic ingredient, and the USDA tried to ban this additive in the 1970s but was vetoed by food manufacturers, who complained that they had no alternative for preserving packaged meat products. Why does the industry still use it? Simple; this chemical just happens to turn meats bright red. It's actually a colour fixer, and it makes old, dead meats appear fresh and vibrant. It is found in: hot dogs, bacon, ham, luncheon meat, cured meats, corned beef, smoked fish or any other type of processed meat.

- BHA and BHT (E320)
BHA (butylated hydroxyanisole) and BHT (butylated hydroxytoluene) are preservatives found in cereals, chewing

gum, potato chips and vegetable oils. This common preservative keeps foods from changing colour, changing flavour or becoming rancid. They affect the neurological system of the brain, alter behaviour and have potential to cause cancer. BHA and BHT are oxidants which form cancer–causing reactive compounds in your body. They are found in: potato chips, gum, cereal, frozen sausages, enriched rice, lard, shortening, candy and jello.

- Sulphur Dioxide (E220)
  Sulphur additives are toxic and in the United States of America the Federal Drugs Administration have prohibited their use on raw fruit and vegetables. Adverse reactions include bronchial problems (particularly in those prone to asthma), hypotension (low blood pressure), flushing and tingling sensations or anaphylactic shock. It also destroys vitamins B1 and E. Not recommended for consumption by children. The International Labour Organisation advises avoidance of E220 if you suffer from conjunctivitis, bronchitis, emphysema, bronchial asthma or cardiovascular disease. It is found in: beer, soft drinks, dried fruit, juices, cordials, wine, vinegar and potato products.

- Potassium Bromate
  An additive used to increase volume in some white flour, breads and rolls, potassium bromate is known to cause cancer in animals. Even small amounts in bread can create problems for humans. It is found in breads.

Appendix 8 — Theta Super Cilver

The three main grades of processed silver (cilver)are:

Colloidal Silver — Silver that is electronically processed into a fine state of subdivision that is suspended in liquid and due to the electronic charge holds its individual character and settles very slowly.

Ionic Silver — Electronically processed silver that is broken down into a free electron (or subatomic particle) that exists in solution.

"SUPER CILVER" — Cilver that has been electronically pushed into a state where it develops a self perpetuating pulse rate that is eternal in nature and pulses too rapidly for individual recording. One definition given by a noted physicist, Robert C. Beck, is that the cilver when processed by this method loses its identity as a trace element i.e. is not identified as a 'particle' and acts more like a gas. Other research professionals have tested this cilver and found the exact same thing. It is etheric in nature, but carries the signature of the element cilver. Super cilver has been extensively tested on literally tens of thousands of people with impressive success.

Colloidal and Ionic Silver are in a three dimensional physical form and take up space. Even if so small that they do not harmfully build up in the body, there is a second problem. One of the world's leading physicists, considered to be the father of electro–medicine today, Robert C. Beck, tested these three forms of silver for penetrability. He found that all forms of Colloidal and Ionic silver had 5%–6% effectiveness for penetrating certain membranes. When he tested Super Cilver he was astonished to see 100% penetration.

Another major distinction between Super Cilver and all others is that due to its energetic and etheric nature, it doesn't break down. Direct sunlight does not change its composition even after years of exposure.

Silver (cilver) has been used for thousands of years for health care. It is believed to be a systematic disinfectant and works like a secondary immune system. Since silver (cilver) kills only bacteria that is anaerobic or nitrogen breathing, the friendly, aerobic (oxygen–breathing) bacteria in the digestive tract are immune to it.

Appendix 9 — New Protocol to Treat Neuroendocrine Development

- Continue pazopanib (Votrient) 400mg daily (slows down growth of cancer cells and used for patients who have had chemotherapy) and sodium phenylbutyrate
- Add everolimus 10mg every other day orally (slows growth of cancer by inhibiting a protein called MTOR which triggers cancer cells to grow and divide)
- vorinostat 100mg daily orally (chemotherapy drug)
- bortezomib 1.3mg/1 sqm of body surface weekly intravenously (chemotherapy drug)
- Stop the bevacizumab, docetaxel, degarelix, rilutek, tyverb.

Appendix 10 — Chronology

Jan 2004	First apparent symptoms causing visits to doctor followed during the year by regular visits
During 2004	Regular visits to doctor for reduced libido and fatigue
During 2004	Facelift made problem apparent
18 Nov 2004	Diagnosis
Dec 2004.	Began hormone therapy (goserelin)
5 Jan 2005	Radical prostatectomy operation
31 May 2005	First visit to Doctor Hilu
1 July 2005	Last dose of goserelin
21 Nov 2005	First meeting with Professor Oliver
21 Nov 2005	Hormone therapy stopped
Mar 2008	Visit to Alternative Medicine Clinic
April 2008	Cancer became more aggressive–reverted to hormone therapy with new drug flutamideJ
July 2008	Reverted to bicalutamide
Sept 2008	Added goserelin
Dec 2008	Added zoledronic acid to help to strengthen bones
April 2009	Visit to Paracelsus Clinic

April 2009	Admitted for pain control (diethylstilbestrol and dexamethasone)
Jun 2009	Again admitted for pain control
Jun 2009	Began oral chemotherapy (chlorambucil and lomustine) which was not effective so it was changed to docetaxel (IV chemotherapy)
Aug 2009	Added carboplatin and shortly after degarelix
Jan 2010	Double-vision and unable to walk far
Mar 2010	Visit to the Cancer Clinic and began taking bevacizumab and other targeted gene therapies
Apr 2010	Osteonecrosis of the jaw
Jun 2010	Break from tablets as sick and not eating
Jul 2010	Combined docetaxel with bevacizumab
Nov 2010	New treatment protocol (Appendix 9)
13 Jan 2011	Joe sadly died

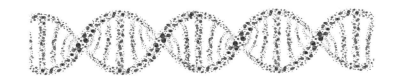

16 - Index

Budwig diet 59, 60
butter 115, 116

C

Cancer Clinic 12, 65, 88, 89, 93, 96, 98, 99, 155, 158, 161, 162, 163, 209
Cancer Decisions 38, 39
Canned and Processed Foods 116
carboplatin 64, 177, 209
carcinogen 111, 133, 117, 122, 123, 177, 187, 202
Cellfood 57, 199
cellular medicine 51, 52, 54, 59, 77, 83
Cesium Chloride 133
chelation therapy 68, 177
chemotherapy 12, 38, 40, 56, 57, 58, 59, 64, 68, 69, 80, 81, 82, 86, 88, 91,
         97, 134, 138, 140, 141, 143, 147, 151, 156, 158, 175, 176, 177, 178,
         179, 181, 207, 209
chlorambucil 64, 177, 209
Chronic Immune Stimulation 74
Chronology 208
clean fifteen 107, 108, 109
clinics 70, 71, 77, 82, 85, 88, 89, 173
Common Food Dyes 120, 203
Cookwear 122
COQ10 56, 57
cores 177
Coy 86, 87
cranio-maxillofacial 95, 151, 155
Crisps 116
Cryosurgery 36
CTC 90, 97, 158, 178

D

darkfield microscopy 51
deep vein thrombosis 99, 163, 164
degarelix 64, 90, 178, 180, 207, 209
demolition 18, 19, 165
detox 141, 146
Detox Electrolysis Footbath 146
detoxification 84, 106, 111, 141, 173
dexamethasone 63, 64, 90, 97, 164, 178, 208
diethylstilbestrol 63, 64, 90, 178, 208

Gonadotropin releasing hormone (GnRH) blocker 180
goserelin 40, 49, 62, 63, 180, 208
GP 29, 30, 54, 95, 97
graviola 56
Greens Drink 127

H

haemoglobin 84, 151, 158, 167
Healthcare at Home 63, 84
HER2 90, 97, 181
HIFU Prostate Treatment 36
High Fructose Corn Syrup 120, 202
hormone therapy 36, 40, 49, 61, 62, 63, 175, 176, 178, 179, 180, 183, 208
hot spots 49
Hulda Clark 142
Hydrogenated Soybean Oil 121
hyperthermia 54, 85, 194, 195

I

Ice Cream 116
IGF–1 119
immune system 9, 10, 28, 51, 52, 53, 56, 58, 68, 72, 74, 81, 82, 85, 96, 101,
        103, 106, 109, 113, 114, 116, 118, 121, 124, 129, 132, 133, 137, 140,
        142, 144, 146, 173, 176, 185, 200, 206
incontinence 35, 37, 38, 42
Iscador Mistletoe Therapy 147

L

lactic acid 86, 185
Lactic acid 86, 185
lapatinib 90, 91, 93, 181
lesions 41, 49, 85, 93, 119, 181
Life Extension 61, 124, 125
Liposomal Vitamin C 131
live blood 51, 67, 68, 69
lomustine 64, 181, 209
Luteinising hormone (LH) blocker 180
lymphovascular invasion 33

M

N

O

P

R

S

T

tyrosine kinase inhibitor 181, 183

V

W

Y

Z

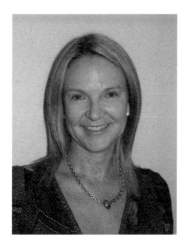

The Author
Julie Romani

Julie began her writing career in 1995 when she successfully self–published 'No Flight of Fancy' which was a best–selling book looking at the subject of pigeon breeding. At that time a well–respected pigeon breeder, her advice helped thousands of pigeon breeders to gain success.

Following the death of her husband from cancer in January 2011, Julie committed herself to the task of writing a book which describes the lessons which they learnt together during their fight against cancer. This book is the result of that endeavour.

The focus of her work is medical and health books with self–help and improvement at their centre.

Today Julie is a successful businesswoman and writer. She lives in West Yorkshire, England, with her family close by.